MCQs and EMQs for the Diploma in Otolaryngology – Head and Neck Surgery

IRFAN SYED
Specialist Registrar, ENT Surgery
South-West Peninsula Deanery
Honorary University Fellow
Peninsula College of Medicine and Dentistry

and

MAHMOOD BHUTTA
Research Fellow
Nuffield Department of Surgery (University of Oxford)
Specialist Registrar, ENT Surgery
Oxford Deanery
Phizackerley Senior Scholar
Balliol College, Oxford

Editorial Advisor
SIMON HICKEY
Consultant ENT Surgeon and Clinical Director in ENT Surgery
Torbay General Hospital, Devon
Training Programme Director
South West Peninsula ENT Rotation

Foreword by
PROFESSOR DAVID HOWARD
Professor of Head & Neck Oncology, Imperial College London
Consultant Head & Neck Surgeon, Charing Cross Hospital, London

Radcliffe Publishing
Oxford • New York

WITHDRAWN
FROM LIBRARY

D1338944

1003263

Radcliffe Publishing Ltd
St Mark's House
Shepherdess Walk
London N1 7BQ
United Kingdom

www.radcliffe-oxford.com

Electronic catalogue and worldwide online ordering facility.

© 2010 Irfan Syed and Mahmood Bhutta

Irfan Syed and Mahmood Bhutta have asserted their right under the Copyright, Designs and Patents Act 1998 to be identified as the author of this work.

All rights reserved. No part of this publication may be reproduced, stored in a retrieval system or transmitted, in any form or by any means, electronic, mechanical, photocopying, recording or otherwise, without the prior permission of the copyright owner.

British Library Cataloguing in Publication Data

A catalogue record for this book is available from the British Library.

ISBN-13: 978 184619 334 7

Typeset by Pindar NZ, Auckland, New Zealand

Contents

Foreword	ix
Preface	x
About the authors	xii

Multiple Choice Questions (MCQs) 1

Otology 3

1	Acute suppurative otitis media	5
2	Otosclerosis	5
3	Retraction pockets of the pars tensa	5
4	Ménière disease	7
5	Complications of ASOM	7
6	Non-organic hearing loss	7
7	Management of BPPV	9
8	Pinna	9
9	Cholesteatoma	9
10	Noise-induced hearing loss	11
11	Otitis externa	11
12	Vestibular schwannoma	11
13	Otalgia	13
14	Tympanic membrane	13
15	Ototoxic drugs	13
16	Pure-tone audiogram	15
17	Nystagmus	15
18	Complications of grommet insertion	15
19	Recurrent ASOM	17
20	Causes of conductive hearing loss	17
21	Cochlea	17
22	Fractures of the temporal bone	19
23	Tinnitus	19
24	Congenital aural atresia	19
25	Tympanic membrane perforation	21
26	Malignant otitis externa	21

27 Complications of modified radical mastoidectomy   21
28 Tympanometry   23
29 Otoacoustic emissions   23
30 Components of the temporal bone   23
31 Causes of tympanic membrane perforation   25
32 Perilymph fistula   25
33 Sensory supply to the pinna   25
34 Tests of vestibular function   27
35 The Eustachian tube   27
36 Mastoid surgery   27
37 Keratosis obturans   29
38 Masses in the external auditory canal   29
39 Bone-anchored hearing aids (BAHA)   29
40 Negative Rinne test   31
41 Objective tests of hearing   31

Rhinology and laryngology   33

42 Adenoidectomy   35
43 Treatments for allergic rhinitis   35
44 Choanal atresia   35
45 Subglottic stenosis   37
46 Juvenile angiofibroma   37
47 Anatomy of the sphenoid sinus   37
48 Sinonasal tumours   39
49 Septal perforation   39
50 Laryngomalacia   39
51 Laryngeal carcinoma   41
52 Respiratory papillomatosis   41
53 Causes of anosmia   41
54 Cerebrospinal fluid (CSF) rhinorrhoea   43
55 Cartilages of the larynx   43
56 Simple nasal polyps   43
57 Vocal nodules   45
58 Causes of allergic rhinitis   45
59 Epistaxis I   45
60 Tests for allergic rhinitis   47
61 Vocal cord palsy   47
62 Complications of septal surgery   47
63 Cilia of the nasal mucosa   49
64 The nasolacrimal duct   49
65 Reinke's oedema   49
66 Laryngocoele   51

67 The frontal sinus   51
68 Hereditary haemorrhagic telangiectasia   51
69 Septal haematoma   55
70 Disorders of smell   55
71 Laryngeal surgery   55
72 The recurrent laryngeal nerve   57
73 Epistaxis II   57

Head and neck   **59**

74   Cause of facial palsy   61
75   Indications for tonsillectomy   61
76   Craniofacial malformations of the airway   61
77   Orbital cellulitis   63
78   Cleft palate   63
79   Midline cystic swelling   63
80   Branches of the facial nerve   65
81   Lymphatic malformation (cystic hygroma)   65
82   Lateral pterygoid muscle   65
83   Temporo-mandibular joint (TMJ)   67
84   Branches of the external carotid artery   67
85   Parotid pleomorphic adenoma   67
86   Oesophageal perforation   69
87   Anterior triangle of the neck   69
88   Mandibular division of the trigeminal nerve   69
89   Posterior triangle of the neck   71
90   Warthin's tumour   71
91   Complications of facial palsy   71
92   Hypopharyngeal carcinoma   73
93   Oral cavity carcinoma   73
94   The submandibular gland   73
95   The tongue   75
96   Papillary adenocarcinoma of the thyroid   75
97   Follicular adenocarcinoma of the thyroid   75
98   Parotid surgery   77
99   Anaplastic carcinoma of the thyroid   77
100 Complications of tracheostomy   77
101 Indications for tracheostomy   79
102 Risk factors for thyroid cancer   79
103 Post-operative chylous fistula   79
104 Facial haemangiomas   81
105 Complications of endotracheal intubation   81
106 Complications of radiotherapy to the head and neck   81

107 Branches of the trigeminal nerve   83
108 Tracheomalacia   83
109 Complications of bilateral neck dissection   83
110 Pharyngeal pouch   85
111 Sjögren syndrome   85
112 The pterygopalatine fossa   85
113 Oral leucoplakia   87
114 The hypoglossal nerve   87
115 Thyroid eye disease   87
116 The glossopharyngeal nerve   89
117 The infratemporal fossa   89
118 Neck injuries   89
119 The thyroid gland   91
120 Salivary calculi   91
121 Barrett's oesophagus   91
122 Branchial cysts   93
123 Parathyroid glands   93

Miscellaneous   **95**

124 Branchial arch derivatives   97
125 Lasers   97
126 Malignant melanoma   97
127 Fine-needle aspiration cytology   99
128 Associations of cigarette smoking   99
129 Obstructive sleep apnoea   99
130 Basal-cell carcinoma   101
131 Risk factors for oesophageal carcinoma   101
132 ENT complications of haematoma   101
133 Evidence-based medicine   103
134 Local anaesthetics   103
135 Wound healing   103
136 Statistical tests   105
137 Surgical sutures   105
138 Consent   105
139 Autoimmune disease   109
140 Orbital blow-out fractures   109
141 Histopathological features of laryngopharyngeal carcinoma   109
142 Chemotherapeutic agents   111
143 Hypovolaemic shock   111
144 The normal infant   111
145 Steroids   113
146 Facial plastics   113

147 Wegener's granulomatosis   113
148 Down syndrome   115
149 Clinical trials   115
150 Imaging   115

Extended Matching Questions (EMQs)   117

Otology   119

    1 Sensorineural hearing loss   121
    2 Conductive hearing loss   121
    3 Dizziness   123
    4 Audiological investigations   123
    5 Syndromic hearing loss   125
    6 Treatment of hearing loss   125
    7 Otalgia   127
    8 Tuning fork tests   127
    9 Hearing aids   129
   10 Congenital hearing loss   129
   11 Tinnitus   131
   12 Management of ear disease   131

Rhinology and laryngology   133

   13 Control of epistaxis   135
   14 Nasal obstruction   135
   15 Rhinorrhoea   137
   16 Staging of laryngeal carcinoma   137
   17 The hoarse voice   139
   18 Acute stridor   139
   19 Throat pain   141
   20 Sinus anatomy   141
   21 Airway management   143
   22 Rhinitis   143
   23 Epistaxis   145

Head and neck   147

   24 Neck dissection   149
   25 Dysphagia   149
   26 Paediatric neck masses   151
   27 Management of thyroid masses   151
   28 Adult neck masses   153
   29 Nerves of the head and neck   153
   30 Nerve injuries in head and neck surgery   155

31 Complications of head and neck surgery   155
32 Vessels of the head and neck   157
33 Salivary gland tumours   157
34 Skull foramina   159
35 Staging of head and neck cancer   159

Miscellaneous   **161**

36 Surgical complications   163
37 Paediatric airway   163
38 Cranial nerve function   165
39 Classes of immunoglobulin   165
40 Thyroid cytology   167
41 Pharyngeal (branchial) arches   167
42 Management of foreign bodies   169
43 Radiological imaging   169
44 Microbial pathogens   171
45 Complications of infection   171
46 ENT manifestations of systemic disease   173
47 Surgical incisions   173
48 Statistical terms   175
49 Endocrine function   175
50 Post-operative investigations   177

Index   **179**

Foreword

The authors of this significant book are no strangers to the subject of MCQs and EMQs, as both have a longstanding interest, and Irfan Syed produced a comprehensive book on EMQs in clinical medicine while still a PRHO in 2004. This new, wide-ranging book presents MCQs and EMQs covering a huge variety of topics in otorhinolaryngology and head and neck surgery, which have direct relevance to clinical practice.

Although MCQs have been developed and increasingly used in examinations since the 1970s, EMQs are becoming a more common form of questioning in both undergraduate and postgraduate examinations. This makes the book applicable to medical students and trainee doctors in general practice as well as in ENT and related head and neck disciplines such as neurology and neurosurgery.

Each question is followed by the correct answer and a clear and concise explanation. Indeed, it is the quality of this additional information that makes this book stand out from its competitors. It provides the student with experience and examination technique in answering these questions, but additionally it is a teaching volume in its own right. It is a credit to its enthusiastic and very competent young teachers in its content, design and clarity, and is another excellent contribution to our thriving specialty.

Professor David Howard
Professor of Head & Neck Oncology, Imperial College London
Consultant Head & Neck Surgeon, Charing Cross Hospital, London
January 2010

Preface

The Diploma in Otolaryngology – Head and Neck Surgery (DOHNS) became an intercollegiate examination in April 2008. In addition, this qualification may now be used towards obtaining membership of any of the surgical colleges of Great Britain. The examination has evolved to fit its new role, and we felt that there was a lack of up-to-date material available for candidates preparing for the written component.

In *MCQs and EMQs for the Diploma in Otolaryngology – Head and Neck Surgery* we aim to fulfil this need. We have drawn upon our previous experience as candidates for this examination, and have tried to focus on topics that are likely to be examined. Each answer is accompanied by an explanation using current evidence-based research wherever possible. We are grateful to Mr Simon Hickey for editorial advice and corrections, but we take responsibility for any errors that remain. We ask readers to contact us with any errors that they detect, so that these may be corrected in future editions.

Good luck with the exam!

Irfan Syed
Mahmood Bhutta
January 2010

For Mum and Dad
I.S.

For A, A and A.
M.B.

About the authors

Irfan Syed is a Specialist Registrar in ENT Surgery in the South West Deanery, and Honorary University Fellow at the Peninsula College of Medicine and Dentistry. His interest in medical education has led to the publication of two previous successful revision textbooks for undergraduate medical students. He has been involved in undergraduate teaching at University College London, and in anatomy demonstrating at Oxford Medical School.

He is on the course faculty for the 'Practical Revision Course for the DO-HNS' at the Royal National Throat, Nose and Ear Hospital, London, and for the 'Introduction to ENT Course' at Torbay Hospital, Devon.

Mahmood Bhutta is currently a research fellow at the University of Oxford, Phizackerley Senior Scholar at Balliol College, Oxford and a Specialist Registrar in ENT in the Oxford Deanery. He has a long-standing interest in teaching. He was previously anatomy demonstrator at the University of Cambridge, has authored a video guide to the ENT examination for medical students at the GKT School of Medicine (King's College London), and has organised a national course to introduce junior doctors to the ENT specialty. His research interests are the aetiology and genetics of otitis media. He is also a founding member of the British Medical Association's Medical Fair and Ethical Trade Group.

Simon Hickey is Consultant ENT Surgeon and Clinical Director in ENT Surgery at Torbay General Hospital, Devon. He is the current Training Programme Director of the South West Peninsula ENT Rotation, and Chair of the National Association of Programme Directors in ENT Surgery. He has a long-standing interest in teaching and the ENT Surgery curriculum, and has been a question setter for the final intercollegiate FRCS examination

BMA

BMA Library

BMA House, Tavistock Square, London WC1H 9JP

British Medical Association
BMA House
Tavistock Square
London
WC1H 9JP

CERTIFICATE OF POSTAGE RECEIPT to be obtained and retained. You are liable for any lost items.

Multiple Choice Questions (MCQs)

Otology

1. Pathogens commonly implicated in acute suppurative otitis media include:
   - *Streptococcus pyogenes*
   - *Haemophilus influenzae*
   - Respiratory syncytial virus
   - Norwalk virus
   - *Moraxella catarrhalis*

2. Otosclerosis:
   - Is a bony overgrowth of the stapes crurae
   - Affects men more than women
   - May be caused by the herpes virus
   - May cause taste disturbance
   - May be managed with a hearing aid

3. Retraction pockets of the pars tensa:
   - May be classified by the Sadé grading system
   - May cause a conductive hearing loss
   - Are associated with Ehlers–Danlos syndrome
   - Are associated with osteogenesis imperfecta
   - Are associated with previous insertion of a ventilation tube

1.   Answers: TTTFT

Streptococcus pyogenes, *Haemophilus influenzae* and *Moraxella catarrhalis* are together cultured from around two-thirds of cases of acute suppurative otitis media. Acute otitis media is preceded by a viral infection in 80–85% of cases, and the most common virus is respiratory syncytial virus. Norwalk viruses cause gastroenteritis.

2.   Answers: FFFFT

Otosclerosis is a genetically mediated metabolic bone disease of uncertain aetiology that affects the otic capsule, typically causing fixation of the stapes footplate. It does not affect the stapes crurae. Although some studies have suggested that women are affected more than men, large-scale studies of temporal bones have shown equal prevalence, and the reported sex difference may be a reflection of gender differences in severity of disease or consultation rates. Measles virus has been found in otosclerotic foci, but there is no evidence to suggest that the herpes virus is involved (although it may be implicated in idiopathic facial palsy). Otosclerosis does not cause taste disturbance, but surgery for the disease may disrupt the chorda tympani nerve, resulting in such a symptom. A hearing aid is a conservative approach to management.

3.   Answers: TTFFT

Sadé has graded retractions of the pars tensa of the tympanic membrane in four stages (1. mild retraction; 2, on to the incus or stapes; 3, touching the promontory; 4, adhered to the promontory). Retraction pockets can cause a conductive hearing loss either through associated erosion of the ossicles or through a lack of aeration around the ossicles. There is no recognised association with the genetic collagen disorders Ehlers–Danlos syndrome and osteogenesis imperfecta. Retraction may occur at the site of previous ventilation tube placement, and there is also an association with a history of chronic otitis media with effusion.

4. Ménière disease:
   - Usually presents in adolescence
   - Is bilateral in two-thirds of cases
   - May be treated by injection of gentamicin into the middle ear
   - Is typically associated with a mid-frequency sensorineural hearing loss
   - Aural fullness is a well-recognised feature

5. Recognised complications of acute suppurative otitis media include:
   - Temporal lobe abscess
   - VIIth cranial nerve palsy
   - VIth cranial nerve palsy
   - Bartholin's abscess
   - Cholesterol cyst/granuloma

6. Non-organic hearing loss:
   - May be diagnosed with Stenger test
   - Is sometimes due to inactive chronic suppurative otitis media
   - May present in childhood
   - Is associated with attempts at financial gain
   - Is best managed with a hearing aid

4.   Answers: FFTTT

Ménière disease presents with attacks of vertigo that are associated with otological symptoms of tinnitus, hearing loss and aural fullness. It usually presents in the 40–60 years age group, and is bilateral in around 20% of cases. Intratympanic gentamicin treatment can be used to treat unilateral Ménière disease, especially if there is little remaining audiological function. The audiogram typically shows a mid-frequency hearing loss.

5.   Answers: TTTFT

Acute suppurative otitis media may cause a temporal lobe abscess by local spread through the tegmen. It may also cause dysfunction of the intratympanic section of the facial nerve, especially if it is dehiscent. If infection spreads to the medial part of the temporal bone, it will cause petrous apicitis, which may present as Gradenigo syndrome (pain in the distribution of the ophthalmic branch of the trigeminal nerve and VIth nerve palsy). If infection spreads along the sternomastoid muscle, it may present anterior to this muscle as a Bezold's abscess (Bartholin's abscess is an abscess of the vulva). There may be haemorrhage in suppurative otitis media, and the cholesterol from membranes of red blood cells may then form a cystic mass, often erroneously termed a cholesterol granuloma.

6.   Answers: TFTTF

Non-organic hearing loss is feigned hearing loss. In adults it is often for financial gain, whereas in children it is often a means of excusing poor school performance. It is by definition not due to any ear disease. Stenger test can be used for diagnosis in non-organic unilateral hearing loss. A pure tone of the same frequency is presented to each ear, but at different levels. In normal individuals such noise is believed to be coming from a single source – the louder one. Individuals who feign hearing loss should have the louder pure tone played to the supposed poorly hearing ear. The individual will then state that they hear nothing, whereas if their hearing loss were real they would actually hear the quieter tone in the good ear. Management does not require a hearing aid, as there is no actual hearing loss.

7. Treatment options for benign paroxysmal positional vertigo (BPPV) include:
   - Unterberger testing
   - Betahistine
   - Politzer manoeuvre
   - Epley manoeuvre
   - Endolymphatic sac decompression

8. The pinna:
   - Helps to localise sound
   - Is usually absent in Treacher–Collins syndrome
   - Is derived from the first pharyngeal pouch
   - Grows by endochondral ossification
   - Is affected in relapsing polychondritis

9. Cholesteatoma:
   - May be congenital
   - Is associated with Niemann–Pick disease
   - Contains cholesterol-rich squamous cells
   - May cause sensorineural hearing loss
   - Can activate osteoclasts

7. Answers: FFFTF

BPPV is a disorder characterised by an abnormal sensation of movement elicited by certain movements. It is thought to be caused by the presence of debris in the semicircular canals, usually the posterior semicircular canal. Medication is rarely effective, and betahistine has no role. Unterberger testing is a method of diagnosis of vestibular disorders, not a treatment. The Epley manoeuvre can reposition debris and abolish symptoms. In resistant cases singular nerve section may be warranted. Endolymphatic sac surgery is used in the treatment of Ménière disease.

8. Answers: TFFFT

The pinna helps to localise sound and is embryologically derived from the six hillocks of Hiss, which are outgrowths from the first and second pharyngeal arches (not the pharyngeal pouch). In first arch malformations such as Treacher–Collins syndrome the pinna may be low-set and small, but it is usually present. It does not ossify, so it does not grow by endo-chondral ossification. Relapsing polychondritis is a rare condition that mainly affects the pinna, nasal skeleton and laryngo-tracheobronchial tree. The cause of polychondritis is uncertain, but it is probably autoimmune.

9. Answers: TFFTT

Cholesteatoma is a mass of keratinising squamous epithelium in the middle ear cleft. The term is a misnomer, as it does not contain excess cholesterol and is not a neoplasm. In advanced disease it may activate osteoclasts to cause ossicular erosion, often of the scutum or the ossicles. In very advanced disease there can be erosion into the cochlea, causing sensorineural hearing loss. Niemann–Pick disease is a lysosomal storage disease that is unrelated to cholesteatoma.

10. Noise-induced hearing loss:
- Affects the basal turn of the cochlea more than the apical turn
- May be caused by meningococcal infection
- Shows genetic variation in susceptibility
- Is a recognised occupational disease under UK legislation
- May be a cause of unilateral tinnitus

11. Otitis externa:
- Is a recognised cause of facial palsy
- May be due to otitis media
- May lead to malignancy of the squamous epithelium of the external ear
- May be caused by topical antibiotic drops
- Swimming is a risk factor

12. Vestibular schwannoma (acoustic neuroma):
- Affects men as often as women
- May present with sudden hearing loss
- Magnetic resonance imaging is the best investigation for imaging
- May be treated with chemoradiotherapy in selected cases
- Is increased in people with neurofibromatosis type 2

10. Answers: TFTTT

Noise exposure can cause irreversible damage to the outer hair cells of the cochlea, particularly those that respond to noises in the 4–6 kHz frequency range (towards the basal turn of the cochlea). There is genetic variation in susceptibility. Meningococcal infection can also cause hearing loss, but this is a separate pathology to noise-induced damage. Tinnitus is encountered frequently in noise-induced hearing loss, and may be unilateral or bilateral. Legislation to protect UK employees from noise exposure may be found in the Health and Safety at Work Act 1974.

11. Answers: TTTTT

Otitis externa may be due to systemic dermal conditions (such as psoriasis), topical hypersensitivity (including a hypersensitive reaction to antibiotic ear drops), or infection (bacterial, fungal or viral). Infective otitis externa is also known as 'swimmer's ear', and humidity is a risk factor in its development. Otitis externa sometimes occurs secondary to discharge from the middle ear, and it is prudent to visualise the tympanic membrane at some point in all patients with otitis externa. Rarely, and particularly in individuals with diabetes, infection may spread into the temporal bone and cause cranial nerve palsies. Very rarely, chronically inflamed external ear squamous epithelium can undergo malignant change.

12. Answers: TTTFT

Vestibular schwannoma is a benign neoplasm of uncertain aetiology that most often affects the superior vestibular nerve. It has an equal gender incidence, but is much more common in individuals with neurofibromatosis type 2, in whom it may be bilateral. It may present with unilateral hearing loss, unilateral tinnitus or sudden unilateral hearing loss. It is best imaged with MRI, and may be treated conservatively, or with radiotherapy or surgery.

13. Recognised causes of otalgia include:
    • Otosclerosis
    • Herpes zoster infection
    • Tonsillar carcinoma
    • Temporo-mandibular joint dysfunction
    • Cervical spondylosis with impingement on the C1 spinal root

14. The tympanic membrane:
    • Is divided into the pars tensa and pars flaccida
    • Is composed of mostly squamous epithelium
    • Is angulated antero-inferiorly
    • May perforate in chronic otitis media with effusion
    • Is embryologically derived from the hillocks of Hiss

15. Ototoxic drugs include:
    • Cisplatin
    • Gentamicin
    • Azithromycin
    • Amikacin
    • Omeprazole

13. Answers: FTTTF

Otalgia may be due to local disease such as otitis media (especially suppurative), otitis externa or trauma to the pinna. Shingles (herpes zoster) is another local cause. However, otosclerosis does not cause otalgia. Otalgia may also be due to referred sources, especially from the glossopharyngeal nerve (e.g. in tonsillar carcinoma or tonsillitis). Other sources of referred otalgia include dental or temporo-mandibular disease, carcinoma of the larynx or hypopharynx, and spinal disease impinging upon the C2 or C3 nerve root. The C1 root does not have any cutaneous branches.

14. Answers: TFTFF

The tympanic membrane has two parts: the superior pars flaccida and the inferior pars tensa. It is angulated antero-inferiorly. It is one of the few structures that are composed of all three embryonic germ cell layers, and so has an ectodermal epithelial layer, a mesodermal fibrous layer and an endodermal mucosal layer. It is embryologically derived from the first pharyngeal cleft, arch and pouch, but not from the hillocks of Hiss, which form the pinna. The tympanic membrane may perforate in acute or chronic suppurative otitis media, but this is not a feature of otitis media with effusion.

15. Answers: TTFTF

Drugs commonly recognised as causing ototoxicity are the platinum-based chemotherapeutic agents (e.g. carboplatin, cisplatin) and certain antibiotics (e.g. amikacin, gentamicin, neomycin, streptomycin). Toxicity is dose dependent, but is also determined by genetic factors. Macrolides, cephalosporins and penicillins are, in general, safe.

16. The pure-tone audiogram:
    - Measures hearing in the 2000–9000 Hz range
    - Uses the symbol 'X' to represent air conduction thresholds in the left ear
    - Is a logarithmic assessment of the sound-pressure level
    - Requires a soundproof booth
    - Is an objective assessment of hearing

17. Nystagmus:
    - In the UK is named according to the fast phase of the response
    - Is first degree if present on forward gaze
    - If vertical is indicative of central nervous system pathology
    - May be inherited
    - Is a sign of giant-cell arteritis

18. Complications of grommet (ventilation tube) insertion include:
    - Infection
    - Permanent perforation of the tympanic membrane
    - Facial palsy
    - Tympanic membrane atelectasis
    - Ménière disease

16. Answers: FTTTF

A pure-tone audiogram (PTA) measures hearing thresholds in the range 250–8000 Hz in a soundproof booth. It is measured on the dB HL scale, which is a logarithmic conversion of the sound-pressure level. The PTA is a subjective assessment of hearing, as it requires the subject to respond. Auditory brainstem response is an objective measure of hearing thresholds. British Society of Audiology recommended audiogram symbols are shown below:

X air conduction threshold left ear
O air conduction threshold right ear
Δ unmasked bone conduction
] masked bone conduction left ear
[masked bone conduction right ear

17. Answers: TFTTF

Nystagmus is a periodic rhythmic ocular oscillation. It may be congenital with a hereditary component, or acquired (due to a variety of disorders). It has a slow phase representing gradual loss of fixation, with a rapid phase to restore that fixation. In the UK it is named according to the fast phase. First-degree nystagmus is present only when the eyes deviate towards the direction of the fast phase of the nystagmus. Second-degree nystagmus is present when the patient looks straight ahead. Third-degree nystagmus is present in all directions of gaze. Direction of nystagmus may be horizontal, vertical or torsional, and vertical nystagmus is generally indicative of a central lesion. Visual changes may occur in giant-cell arteritis affecting the ophthalmic artery, but nystagmus is not a typical feature.

18. Answers: TTFTF

Around 20% of grommets will be associated with infection, and around 1–2% will end up with a permanent perforation. When the tympanic membrane has healed, the healed section may be atelectatic and/or retracted. Facial palsy should not occur with grommet insertion. Grommet insertion is a (controversial) treatment for Ménière disease, not a cause of it.

19. Recurrent acute suppurative otitis media:
    • Is most common between the ages of 4 and 6 years
    • May be a cause of sensorineural hearing loss
    • May be associated with reduced immunoglobulin A levels
    • May cause myringosclerosis
    • Is more common in individuals with cystic fibrosis

20. Causes of conductive hearing loss include:
    • Osteogenesis imperfecta
    • Tympanic membrane retraction
    • Tympanosclerosis
    • Cytomegalovirus
    • Nasopharyngeal carcinoma

21. The cochlea:
    • Has three and a half turns
    • Receives its blood supply from the internal carotid artery
    • The scala media contains perilymph
    • Is elongated in Mondini dysplasia
    • Displays tonotopic structure

19. Answers: FTTTF

Recurrent acute suppurative otitis media is most common at the age of 2 years, probably due to immunological immaturity. It is associated with reduced IgA levels in some cases. It can lead to patches of calcium deposition in the tympanic membrane (myringosclerosis), although the pathophysiological mechanism of such changes is uncertain. It can also cause cochlear damage, probably due to translocation of toxins across the round window. There is no association with cystic fibrosis.

20. Answers: TTTFT

Conductive hearing loss can be caused by obstruction of the external auditory canal, or by disease of the middle ear. Middle ear pathology as a cause of conductive hearing loss may be an effusion replacing the normally gaseous middle ear environment, or a problem with the ossicles. A middle ear effusion is common in childhood, but rare in adults. A unilateral effusion in adulthood may be the first sign of nasopharyngeal carcinoma. Tympanosclerosis rarely causes conductive hearing loss, but if extensive it can cause ossicular fixation. Tympanic membrane retraction can lead to ossicular erosion, typically of the long process of the incus, or in severe retractions, a loss of middle ear aeration. Patients with osteogenesis imperfecta suffer from pathological fractures, including fractures of the ossicles. Cytomegalovirus infection during the first trimester can cause prenatal sensorineural hearing loss.

21. Answers: FFFFT

The cochlea has two and a half turns, and Mondini dysplasia is a defect that causes fewer turns. The cochlea receives its blood supply from the internal labyrinthine artery, which is a branch of the basilar artery (vertebral artery). It has three sections, namely the scala media (cochlear duct) containing endolymph, and the scala vestibuli and scala tympani containing perilymph. The basilar membrane of the cochlea displays tonotopy – that is, a spatial arrangement of response to different frequencies of sound.

22. Fractures of the temporal bone may cause:
    - Delayed facial weakness
    - External auditory canal stenosis
    - Weakness of the tongue
    - Conductive hearing loss
    - Sensorineural hearing loss

23. Tinnitus:
    - May be caused by palatal myoclonus
    - Is very rare in children
    - May be treated with white noise
    - Is frequent in sufferers of benign paroxysmal positional vertigo
    - If unilateral is likely to be due to vestibular schwannoma (acoustic neuroma)

24. Congenital aural atresia:
    - Is usually associated with cochlear malformation
    - May be found in Moebius syndrome
    - Is bilateral in most cases
    - Is associated with cleft palate
    - May be treated with mitomycin C

22. Answers: TTFTT

Fracture of the temporal bone occurs following significant head injury, usually resulting from road traffic accidents. The displaced bone fragments may disrupt the contours of the external auditory canal, disrupt the ossicles, fracture the cochlea or damage the facial nerve. Management of the facial nerve is important to reduce morbidity. Immediate total facial weakness suggests a transection of the nerve (which requires exploration), whereas delayed onset or incomplete facial weakness suggests physiological disruption of the nerve (which is treated conservatively). Disruption of the facial nerve can lead to altered taste sensation in the tongue, but not altered motor function of the tongue.

23. Answers: TFTFF

Tinnitus is the perception of noise not generated in the external environment. Objective causes include arteriovenous malformations, glomus tumours and palatal myoclonus. Vestibular schwannoma can also cause unilateral tinnitus, but only around 1% of those with unilateral tinnitus will have a vestibular schwannoma. Tinnitus is not uncommon in childhood, but is under-reported. It is not a characteristic of benign positional paroxysmal vertigo, and the combination of vertigo with tinnitus suggests other pathology. Treatments include retraining therapies and white-noise generators ('maskers').

24. Answers: FTFTF

Congenital aural atresia is an embryonic failure of the development of the middle and external ear. Although they develop separately, both the middle ear and external ear are derived from the first and second pharyngeal arches, which explains the associated malformations. The vast majority of cases are not associated with cochlear malformation (the cochlea has a separate embryological origin), but it is important to demonstrate good cochlear function before embarking upon surgery to overcome conductive hearing loss. The malformation is unilateral in around 80% of cases. There is an association with malformation of the facial nerve (e.g. Moebius syndrome) but also with cleft palate (e.g. in Treacher–Collins syndrome), urogenital malformation and cardiovascular malformation. Treatment is conservative, using bone-anchored hearing aids or surgical repair, usually utilising costal cartilage to fashion a pinna.

25. Tympanic membrane perforation:
- Can be caused by acute suppurative otitis media
- May be repaired using cartilage
- May be associated with a hearing loss of up to 80 dB
- Can occur following grommet (ventilation tube) surgery
- Will give a Jerger type C tympanogram

26. Malignant otitis externa:
- Is more common in diabetics
- Often causes hypoglossal nerve palsy
- Is often treated with radiotherapy
- Usually occurs in children
- CT scanning can aid management

27. Complications of modified radical mastoidectomy include:
- Conductive hearing loss
- Sensorineural hearing loss
- Dysphagia
- Taste disturbance
- Facial neuroma

25. Answers: TTFTF

The most common cause of tympanic membrane perforation is acute suppurative otitis media, but it can also be caused by trauma (including barotrauma) or previous grommet surgery. Repair of the tympanic membrane (myringoplasty) can be achieved using a variety of substances to provide a 'scaffold' for repair, but the use of cartilage is gaining increasing popularity. Tympanic membrane perforations tend to cause a mild conductive hearing loss, but even a maximal conductive hearing loss will give thresholds of 60 dB. A perforation will cause a type B (flat) tympanogram with a large ear canal volume.

26. Answers: TFFFT

Malignant otitis externa occurs when infection spreads from the external auditory canal to the temporal bone. Spread of infection can cause dysfunction of cranial nerves, especially the facial nerve, but the hypoglossal nerve is not in anatomical proximity and so is rarely affected. The disease usually occurs in adults who are diabetic or immunocompromised. It can also occur in those who have previously had radiotherapy to this area. CT of the temporal bones can show the extent of the disease. Treatment is with prolonged systemic antibiotics and sometimes local surgical debridement.

27. Answers: TTFTF

Mastoidectomy can lead to damage to the ossicles (usually dislocation), causing conductive hearing loss, as well as damage to the cochlea, causing sensorineural hearing loss. Taste disturbance is not infrequent, due to damage to or transection of the chorda tympani, but it often recovers or passes unnoticed. Dysphagia can result from damage to the nerve fibres destined for the pharyngeal plexus, but these do not run through the middle ear. Facial neuroma is a rare entity of uncertain cause, but there is no association with previous middle ear surgery.

28. Tympanometry:
- Requires an airtight seal
- Is typically Jerger type A in otosclerosis
- Is typically Jerger type C in tympanic membrane perforation
- May be Jerger type B in a newborn child
- Requires a soundproof booth

29. Otoacoustic emissions (OAEs):
- Are generated from the inner hair cells of the cochlea
- May be absent in the presence of middle ear effusion
- Are a useful screen for neonatal hearing loss
- Can be used to diagnose central processing disorders
- Are absent in adults

30. The following anatomical structures are components of the temporal bone:
- Clinoid process
- Mastoid process
- Styloid process
- Medial pterygoid plate
- Zygomatic process

28. Answers: TTFTF

Tympanometry is a measure of acoustic admittance into the middle ear at differing pressures applied to the tympanic membrane by a column of air in the external auditory canal. It is effectively a measure of middle ear pressure. It requires an airtight seal, and although a quiet area is required, a soundproof booth is unnecessary. The tympanogram can broadly be divided into Jerger type A (normal, maximal admittance at atmospheric pressure), Jerger type B (no or little admittance, usually indicative of middle ear effusion or perforation) or Jerger type C (peak admittance at sub-atmospheric pressure, implying low pressure in the middle ear). In otosclerosis the tympanogram is not affected. With a tympanic membrane perforation, the tympanic membrane will not move with a column of air applied lateral to it, causing a Jerger type B tympanogram (it can usually be differentiated from middle ear effusion by the relatively large ear canal volume measured). A Jerger type B tympanogram can also be seen in the newborn child due to the presence of amniotic fluid in the middle ear, which is not infrequent, and probably of no long-term consequence.

29. Answers: FTTFF

Otoacoustic emissions (OAEs) are measures of the electrical activity of the outer hair cells of the cochlea. They are measured by a probe in the external auditory canal, and may be generated spontaneously or in response to sound. They are specific for demonstrating cochlear function, but not sensitive. Any obstruction to the detection of these emissions, such as a middle ear effusion, may give a false-negative result. In addition, OAEs do not assess processing of sound upstream of the cochlea, and auditory brainstem and cortical response testing is necessary for diagnosis of central processing disorders. As they are cheap, specific and non-invasive, OAEs are used for universal neonatal screening of hearing in the UK and elsewhere. OAEs remain present throughout life.

30. Answers: FTTFT

The mastoid, styloid and zygomatic process are all parts of the temporal bone. The medial pterygoid plate and the clinoid processes are components of the sphenoid.

31. Recognised causes of tympanic membrane perforation include:
- Explosion injuries
- Human papilloma virus
- *Streptococcus pneumoniae*
- *Haemophilus influenzae*
- *Mycobacterium tuberculosis*

32. Perilymph fistula:
- Is a cause of unexpected sensorineural loss in children
- May follow head trauma
- Most often arises from the round window
- Diving is contraindicated
- High-definition CT scan may be useful for diagnosis

33. The sensory supply to the pinna includes contributions from:
- C1 nerve fibres
- The vagus (X) nerve
- The spinal accessory (XI) nerve
- The trigeminal (V) nerve
- The ansa cervicalis

31.   Answers: TFTTT

The most common cause of tympanic membrane perforation is acute otitis media, and the most common bacterial pathogens involved are *Streptococcus pneumoniae* and non-typeable *Haemophilus influenzae*. *Mycobacterium tuberculosis* is a less common cause of perforation, and classically presents with multiple small perforations. Non-infective causes of perforation are traumatic, including barotrauma from diving, air travel or blast injuries. Human papilloma virus does not cause tympanic membrane perforation.

32.   Answers: TTFTT

Perilymph fistula is an abnormal connection between the air-filled middle ear and the fluid-filled inner ear. The two most common sites of weakness are the oval window (60% of cases) and round window niche (20%). Because of this abnormal connection, changes in the middle ear pressure directly affect the inner ear, causing vertigo. Barotrauma and head trauma are the most common causes of perilymph fistulae. Congenital perilymph fistulae are rare, but should be considered in children with an unexplained fluctuating or progressive sensorineural hearing loss. There may be associated middle and inner ear deformities (e.g. Mondini dysplasia or stapes malformation). Diving is contraindicated, as the change in atmospheric pressure could precipitate vertigo underwater. High-resolution CT is the imaging of choice.

33.   Answers: FTFTF

The major sensory supply to the pinna is from the great auricular nerve, which contains C2 and C3 fibres from the cervical plexus. There is no C1 dermatome. The vagus gives an auricular branch to the posterior external auditory canal and pinna (Arnold's nerve). The auriculotemporal branch of the mandibular (V3) nerve also supplies the pinna. The spinal accessory nerve has no sensory component and neither does the ansa cervicalis.

34. The following are tests of vestibular function:
    - CT scan
    - Electronystagmography
    - Tympanometry
    - Unterberger test
    - Caloric testing

35. The Eustachian tube:
    - Is about 5–7 cm in length
    - Opens into the medial wall of the nasopharynx
    - Is cartilaginous along the medial two-thirds
    - Is lined with ciliated epithelium
    - Has a smaller angle to the horizontal plane in children than in adults

36. Mastoid surgery:
    - The main aim of cholesteatoma surgery is to reconstruct ossicular damage
    - In canal-wall-down procedures a low facial ridge is preferable
    - Modified radical mastoidectomy usually requires a second look under general anaesthesia
    - Combined-approach tympanoplasty is the most common canal-wall-down procedure
    - Ossicular reconstruction is possible in both canal-wall-up and canal-wall-down procedures

34. Answers: FTFTT

There are several clinical tests of vestibular function. The Unterberger test involves asking the patient to march up and down on the spot. If there is vestibular hypofunction, the patient will turn to the side of the lesion. Electronystagmography tests the integrity of the vestibulo-ocular reflex by measuring chorio-retinal electrical potential. Normal eye movements are assessed, as well as the response to positional changes and to caloric testing. Caloric testing involves irrigating the external auditory canal with warm or cold water which stimulates the labyrinth. In the normal ear, cold water causes nystagmus to the opposite side to that being irrigated, and warm water causes nystagmus to the same side. Tympanometry is an assessment of tympanic membrane deformation and consequently of middle ear pressure. A CT scan can provide useful anatomical information about the inner ear, but does not provide a functional assessment.

35. Answers: FFTTT

The Eustachian tube is around 36 mm long in adults. It runs forward and medially from the middle ear to the lateral wall of the nasopharynx. The lateral third is bony and joins the medial cartilaginous two-thirds at the isthmus. The tube is lined with respiratory ciliated mucosa. In children the Eustachian tube is shorter and has a smaller angle to the horizontal plane compared with adults. It has been suggested that this anatomical difference accounts for an increased risk of otitis media in children, but this view is controversial.

36. Answers: FTFFT

The main aim of cholesteatoma surgery is to clear disease and prevent the development of further cholesteatoma. Restoration of hearing is a secondary aim, and ossicular reconstruction can always be delayed. Combined-approach tympanoplasty is a 'canal-wall-up' procedure, as the external auditory canal is maintained and the tympanic membrane is in its normal position. In 'canal-wall-down' procedures (e.g. modified radical mastoidectomy), the posterior wall of the external auditory canal is opened into the mastoid to create a single cavity. Ossicular reconstruction is possible with both techniques.

37. Keratosis obturans:
- Is a pre-malignant condition
- Is usually bilateral
- Rarely causes otalgia
- Is associated with widening of the bony canal
- May be managed with simple aural toilet

38. Masses in the external auditory canal:
- Wax impaction is the most common cause of moderate to severe conductive hearing loss
- Wax plugs should be removed with olive oil and careful use of a cotton bud
- Exostoses are associated with a history of swimming in cold water
- Osteomas usually require surgical excision
- A button battery in the ear should be treated with topical antibiotics prior to removal

39. Bone-anchored hearing aids (BAHA):
- Transmit sound directly from the skull to the inner ear
- A gold fixture is used for osseointegration due to its inert properties
- Bilateral canal atresia is an indication for BAHA implantation
- May be useful in patients with severe unilateral hearing loss
- Failure to osseointegrate is the commonest complication of BAHA implantation

37. Answers: FTFTT

Keratosis obturans is the accumulation of large plaques of desquamated keratin in the external auditory canal. The cause of the condition is uncertain. It is usually bilateral and typically presents with severe otalgia, but may also be associated with a conductive hearing loss due to the physical obstruction. The enlarging plug of keratin gives rise to inflammation and increased osteoclast activity, causing canal widening. Management involves aural toilet, which may need to be performed under general anesthetic due to pain. Corticosteroid drops may help to reduce the associated inflammation.

38. Answers: FFTFF

Contrary to popular belief, wax impaction, even with large quantities of wax, is not associated with significant conductive hearing impairment. Olive oil may be used to soften wax and aid microsuction, but cotton buds should never be used, due to the risk of trauma to the external auditory canal and the tympanic membrane. Exostoses are benign bony growths that can be found in the external auditory canal. They are often multiple and associated with chronic exposure to cold water. Osteomas are usually single and located at the bony–cartilaginous border. They do not require surgical excision except in rare instances when they are causing conductive hearing loss or recurrent infection due to water trapping. A button battery in the ear is an emergency that requires immediate removal. Topical eardrops are contraindicated in this situation, as they may cause leakage of alkali from the battery and corrosion of the ear canal.

39. Answers: TFTTF

Bone-anchored hearing aids consist of a titanium implant, an external abutment and a sound processor. Sound is transmitted by bone conduction along the skull to the inner ear, bypassing the external auditory canal and middle ear. Titanium is used for the fixture due to its ability to integrate with bone over time. Bilateral canal atresia is an absolute indication for a bone-anchored hearing aid. Patients with severe unilateral hearing loss may have problems with understanding speech in background noise or in localising sound, and a bone-anchored hearing aid is often a more practical solution than the traditional CROS hearing aids. The more common complications of surgery include crusting and granulation around the operation site. Failure to osseointegrate occurs in less than 1% of cases.

40. The following conditions are associated with a negative Rinne test:
- Presbycusis
- Otosclerosis
- Ménière disease
- Vestibular schwannoma
- Noise-induced hearing loss

41. The following are objective tests of hearing:
- Tympanometry
- Otoacoustic emissions testing
- Brainstem electrical response audiometry
- Pure-tone audiometry
- Speech audiometry

40. Answers: FTFFF

A negative Rinne test is associated with a conductive hearing loss (i.e. bone conduction greater than air conduction). Presbycusis, Ménière disease and vestibular schwannoma are associated with a sensorineural hearing loss.

41. Answers: FTTFF

Hearing tests that require a patient response (e.g. pure-tone audiometry or speech audiometry) are called subjective tests, whereas those that do not require a response (e.g. otoacoustic emission and brainstem response testing) are objective tests. Objective tests are less prone to bias, as patient cooperation is not a factor. They are also particularly useful when subjective tests cannot be used (e.g. in very young children or when a non-organic hearing impairment is suspected). Tympanometry is not a test of hearing.

Rhinology and laryngology

42. Adenoidectomy:
- Is indicated for the treatment of childhood obstructive sleep apnoea
- Reduces the recurrence rate of otitis media with effusion
- May cause a bifid uvula
- Can cause occipito-atlantal subluxation
- May alter dentition

43. Recognised treatments for allergic rhinitis include:
- Oral antihistamines
- Topical steroids
- Oral steroids
- Ultraviolet radiation
- Leukotriene-receptor agonists

44. Choanal atresia:
- May cause neonatal respiratory distress
- Has an incidence of 1 in 500
- Can be unilateral
- Is associated with cardiac defects
- Should be assessed with pre-operative MRI

42.   Answers: TTFFT

Childhood obstructive sleep apnoea is almost always caused by hypertrophy of the lymphatic tissue of Waldeyer's ring, and removal of the tonsils and adenoids is a standard treatment. Several studies have demonstrated that adenoidectomy reduces recurrence of otitis media with effusion in those aged over 4 years, and therefore adenoidectomy is indicated in such cases. Adenoidectomy does not cause a bifid uvula, but the presence of the latter should prompt a search for a submucous cleft palate, because adenoidectomy in the presence of cleft palate could cause palatal incompetence. Atlanto-axial subluxation is a rare consequence of adenoidectomy. There is evidence that adenoidectomy alters the position of the incisor teeth.

43.   Answers: TTTTF

Antihistamines provide relief of symptoms of sneezing and itching, and topical steroids relieve symptoms of nasal blockage. Oral steroids can provide dramatic relief of symptoms, but should be used sparingly because of their systemic side-effects. Ultraviolet radiation has been shown to provide relief of medication-resistant allergic rhinitis, but its long-term side-effects are not known. Leukotriene-receptor antagonists (not agonists), such as montelukast, are licensed for use in individuals with allergic rhinitis and asthma.

44.   Answers: TFTTF

Choanal atresia is a failure of canalisation of the choanae, which affects around 1 in 10 000 births. It is a neonatal emergency that requires intubation, as the neonate is an obligate nasal breather. Two-thirds of cases are unilateral, and half are associated with additional defects. The CHARGE syndrome includes choanal atresia with coloboma of the iris or choroid, heart defects such as atrial septal defect, retarded growth, genitourinary defects, and external, middle or inner ear abnormalities (although all of these abnormalities are rarely present). Pre-operative CT scanning is the most useful imaging technique for demonstrating whether the atresia is bony (90% of cases) or membranous.

45. Subglottic stenosis:
    • May affect the distal trachea
    • Has a genetic predisposition
    • May be treated with an Isshiki thyroplasty
    • Is of Cotton grade IV if the measured luminal diameter is 75% of the expected diameter
    • May be caused by relapsing polychondritis

46. Juvenile angiofibroma:
    • Is more common in female adolescents
    • Is best treated with radiotherapy
    • May present with multiple episodes of epistaxis
    • Diagnosis is confirmed by examination under anaesthesia and biopsy
    • MRI is a useful investigation

47. Anatomy of the sphenoid sinus:
    • It is fully developed at birth
    • It is bordered superiorly by the sella turcica
    • The internal carotid artery runs in its medial wall
    • The Vidian nerve runs below its floor
    • The optic nerve may be found in the lateral wall of the sinus

45.   Answers: FTFFT

Subglottic stenosis (SGS) describes a narrowing of the subglottis (the region between the vocal cords and the lower border of the cricoid). By definition, SGS cannot affect the distal trachea – that would be called tracheal stenosis. The most common cause is endotracheal intubation, but there seems to be no consistent relationship between the number or duration of intubations and the risk of disease. This implies an (unidentified) genetic component. SGS can also be congenital or caused by trauma, relapsing polychondritis, Wegener's granulomatosis or amyloidosis. Grading is usually with the Cotton system, where grade I is obstruction of 0–50% of the normal lumen diameter for that age, grade II is 51–70% obstruction, grade III is 71–99% obstruction and grade IV is 100% obstruction. In severe cases, surgical treatment includes laryngo-tracheal reconstruction. Isshiki thyroplasty is used to treat vocal cord palsy.

46.   Answers: FFTFT

Juvenile angiofibroma is a benign tumour that arises near the sphenopalatine foramen in the lateral nasopharyngeal wall. It occurs almost exclusively in male adolescents. The patient commonly presents with nasal obstruction and recurrent epistaxis. MRI with STIR sequence is a useful investigation for establishing the size and vascularity of the tumour. These tumours should not be biopsied, due to the risk of uncontrollable haemorrhage. The treatment of choice is surgical excision, usually via a mid-facial degloving or cranio-facial approach, depending upon the size and position of the tumour. Some surgeons advocate pre-operative angiography and embolisation of major feeding vessels.

47.   Answers: FTFTT

The sphenoid sinuses remain undeveloped until the age of 3 years, and do not reach full size until the age of 18 years. The sphenoid sinus is bordered superiorly by the sella turcica and pituitary gland. The Vidian canal is found inferior to the sphenoid sinus, and medial to the foramen rotundum. The optic nerve and the internal carotid artery are related to the lateral wall of the sphenoid sinus, and may be dehiscent. They are potentially at risk during endoscopic sphenoidotomy.

48. Sinonasal tumours:
- Usually present early
- Most patients will develop distant metastases
- Inverted papilloma may transform to carcinoma
- There is a strong association with smoking
- Exposure to hardwood dust is associated with squamous-cell carcinoma

49. Septal perforation:
- Iatrogenic injury is a common cause
- Is associated with recreational drug use
- Syphilis is a recognised cause of bony perforation
- Should be biopsied in almost all cases
- Perforations larger than 4 cm in diameter are best treated by surgical closure

50. Laryngomalacia:
- Is more common in males
- Usually presents in the first few days of life
- Has an abnormal cry in most cases
- Stridor is worse in the supine position
- Is associated with an omega-shaped epiglottis

48.   Answers: FFTFF
Due to their position, sinonasal tumours often present late with extensive local disease. Distant metastases are uncommon. Inverted papilloma may undergo malignant transformation to carcinoma. There is no strong association between smoking and sinonasal tumours. Occupational associations include exposure to the dust of hardwoods (for ethmoidal adenocarcinoma) and close contact with the chromium salts/nickel-refining process (for squamous-cell carcinoma).

49.   Answers: TTTFF
Digital trauma from nose picking and iatrogenic injury are the most common causes of septal perforation. The incidence of septal perforation secondary to cocaine use is increasing. Tertiary syphilis should always be considered in the presence of a bony septal perforation. The edge of a septal perforation should be biopsied if there is suspicion of malignancy or a granulomatous disease process. If there is a clear history of iatrogenic injury and the perforation is clean, there is no need for biopsy. Surgical closure of septal perforations is difficult, especially for large perforations. Sometimes septal perforations are better mamnaged by surgical enlargement, as this can also provide symptomatic relief.

50.   Answers: FFFTT
Laryngomalacia is the most common cause of congenital stridor. The condition has an equal sex distribution. It usually presents in the first 2 months of life with squeaky inspiratory noises. The epiglottis is floppy and tends to prolapse into the laryngeal inlet during respiration. In cross-section the epiglottis is often omega-shaped. The stridor is typically worse in the supine position. The cry is usually normal unless there is associated reflux.

51. Laryngeal carcinoma:
- Squamous-cell carcinoma is the most common laryngeal malignancy
- Stridor is a common early presenting symptom
- Pain may be referred to the ear
- Direct examination and biopsy under general anaesthetic are mandatory
- Small tumours can be treated by radiotherapy alone

52. Respiratory papillomatosis:
- Is associated with herpes zoster virus infection
- May result in acute upper airway obstruction
- In adults may undergo malignant transformation
- Small lesions may be treated with radiotherapy
- Laser surgery is usually curative

53. Causes of anosmia include:
- Road traffic accident
- Upper respiratory tract infection
- Holoprosencephaly
- Nasal polyposis
- Kallmann syndrome

51. Answers: TFTTT

Squamous-cell carcinoma is the most common laryngeal malignancy, and usually presents early due to dysphonia. Stridor is a late sign due to impairment of the airway. The vagus and glossopharyngeal nerves have tympanic and auricular branches, so both laryngeal and oropharyngeal malignancies may be associated with otalgia. Early glottic cancer may be treated with radiotherapy or surgical excision.

52. Answers: FTTFF

Respiratory papillomatosis is associated with human papilloma virus infection, in particular the HPV-6 and HPV-11 subtypes. It can cause significant airway obstruction, and may require tracheostomy to secure the airway. CO_2 laser excision is considered by most to be the treatment of choice, and multiple treatments are often required to keep the disease under control. Treatment is not usually curative, and current research is exploring the use of antiviral agents, e.g. cidofovir or vaccines, to try to eradicate local HPV infection.

53. Answers: TTTTT

Anosmia can be caused by obstruction of the olfactory cleft (e.g. due to nasal polyposis) or by problems with the olfactory neurons. Acquired damage to the olfactory nerves can occur as a result of shearing of the olfactory bulb with an anterior skull base fracture (e.g. following RTA) or neurological damage due to viral upper respiratory tract infection. Rare inherited causes of anosmia include Kallmann syndrome, which is a failure of migration of gonadotrophin-releasing hormone neurons that leads to hypogonadism and agenesis or hypoplasia of the olfactory bulb. Holoprosencephaly is caused by failure of development of the prosencephalon (forebrain), and may lead to facial as well as cerebral defects.

54. Cerebrospinal fluid (CSF) rhinorrhoea:
- Can occur following nasal polypectomy
- Can occur following trauma
- When iatrogenic, is more likely in a Keros type III than a Keros type I cribriform plate
- May be treated with beta-2 transferrin
- May cause meningitis

55. The following are cartilages of the larynx:
- Thyroid cartilage
- Cuneiform cartilage
- Trapezoid cartilage
- Cricoid cartilage
- Thyropharyngeal cartilage

56. Simple nasal polyps:
- Are more common in individuals with asthma
- Are typically tender to touch
- Can become malignant
- Are associated with colonic polyps
- May be treated with oral steroids

54. Answers: TTTFT

CSF rhinorrhoea typically occurs following trauma (either a traumatic skull base injury or iatrogenic trauma during nasal or sinus surgery). The Keros system classifies the depth of the olfactory fossa: type 1 is a depth of 1–3 mm, type 2 is a depth of 4–7 mm, and type III is a depth of 8–16 mm. In Keros type III the lateral lamella of the cribriform plate is more likely to be injured. CSF leakage may be diagnosed by the finding of beta-2 transferrin, which is both sensitive and specific. The risk of meningitis is around 10% in the first 3 weeks following traumatic leaks, and around 40% in leaks due to other causes.

55. Answers: TTFTF

The cartilages of the larynx are the thyroid cartilage, the epiglottis, the cricoid and the paired arytenoid, corniculate and cuneiform cartilages.

56. Answers: TFFFT

Nasal polyps are oedematous polypoidal swellings of the nose and paranasal sinuses of uncertain aetiology. They can be associated with asthma and aspirin sensitivity, which is termed 'Samter's triad.' They are insensate, are not associated with polyps at other anatomical sites and are not pre-malignant. However, a pre-malignant polyp such as inverted papilloma can look similar to a simple polyp. Therefore any unilateral nasal polyp should be biopsied. Treatment is with topical or oral steroids, or surgery if steroid treatment fails.

57. Vocal nodules:
- Are more common in women
- Typically occur midway along the vocal cord
- May be treated with speech therapy
- May cause dysphagia
- Are treated with cidofovir in recurrent cases

58. Common allergens that cause allergic rhinitis in the UK include:
- Cat saliva
- Faeces of house dust mite
- Lactose
- Timothy-grass
- Ragweed

59. The following are associated with an increased risk of epistaxis:
- Hereditary haemorrhagic telangiectasia
- High atmospheric pressure
- Polycythaemia vera
- Factor V Leiden
- Facial trauma

57. Answers: TFTFF

Vocal nodules are inflammatory masses that appear following voice strain or abuse (i.e. yelling or shouting). They occur at the junction of the anterior one-third and posterior two-thirds of the vocal cord, where the cords collide with the greatest force. They will cause dysphonia and sometimes painful vocalisation, but dysphagia does not occur. Treatment is with voice rest and speech therapy, or rarely with microlaryngeal excision. Cidofovir may be used for recurrent laryngeal papillomatosis, but not for vocal nodules.

58. Answers: TTFTF

Allergic rhinitis is caused by a type 1 hypersensitivity reaction to inhaled particles that become trapped in the nasal filtration mechanism. The responsible particle may be pollen that is released seasonally, such as that of timothy-grass, rye-grass, birch, etc. Ragweed pollen is a very common cause of seasonal allergic rhinitis worldwide, but rare as a cause in the UK. Perennial rhinitis may be caused by particles from cat saliva (fel d1), dog fur, or faeces of house dust mite (Der f1/Der p1). Food substances such as lactose are very rarely a cause of allergic rhinitis.

59. Answers: TFTFT

Any trauma to the nose can lead to epistaxis, whether through surgery or from other sources. Some disorders are associated with an increased risk of bleeding, including hereditary haemorrhagic telangiectasia (HHT), also known as Osler–Weber–Rendu syndrome, which is due to an abnormality in capillary structure. Haematological disorders such as haemophilia, leukaemia, multiple myeloma, idiopathic thrombocytopaenic purpura and polycythaemia vera also confer an increased risk. Factor V Leiden is an abnormal form of coagulation factor V associated with hypercoagulability. Atmospheric pressure is not clearly associated with risk of epistaxis, although it has been suggested that lower temperatures may be a risk factor, but this is associated with low, not high, atmospheric pressure.

60. The following tests can be useful for elucidating the cause of allergic rhinitis:
- Radio-allergosorbent test (RAST)
- Saccharine test
- Total serum IgE levels
- Skin prick testing
- Acoustic rhinometry

61. Vocal cord palsy:
- Affects the right cord more often than the left
- May be caused by bronchial carcinoma
- Is associated with Budd–Chiari syndrome
- May predispose to pneumonia
- Can be treated with Isshiki type I thyroplasty

62. Recognised complications of submucous resection/septoplasty include:
- Septal perforation
- Polly beak deformity
- Anosmia
- Palatal anaesthesia
- Frey syndrome

60. Answers: TFFTF

Tests commonly used to elucidate the cause of allergic rhinitis are those that measure antigen-specific IgE levels *in vitro*, and those that measure skin response to *in-vivo* antigen challenge. Antigen-specific IgE levels can be measured by the radio-allergosorbent test. This relies on the binding of IgE from the patient's serum to specific allergens, and subsequent demonstration of these with a radiolabelled anti-IgE antibody. An alternative test is the enzyme-linked immunosorbent assay (ELISA), which uses an enzyme-activated marker instead of a radioactive one. Measurement of total IgE levels is insufficiently specific to allow diagnosis of the cause of the allergic response. *In-vivo* testing, such as skin prick tests, involves injection of an antigen into the upper layers of the skin and comparison of the response to positive (histamine) and negative (e.g. glycerin) controls after 20 minutes. The saccharine test is a test of ciliary function, and acoustic rhinometry is a measure of nasal cross-sectional area and volume. Neither has any value in determining the cause of allergic rhinitis.

61. Answers: FTFTT

Vocal cord palsy affects the left vocal cord more often than the right because of the longer course of the left recurrent laryngeal nerve. It can be caused by a disorder of the cord itself, such as a laryngeal carcinoma, or by dysfunction of the recurrent laryngeal nerve. The latter may be due to trauma (including iatrogenic trauma following thoracic or thyroid surgery), malignancy in the thorax, thyroid, larynx or oesophagus, or neurological disorders affecting motor nerves or the brainstem. Bilateral vocal cord palsy may be caused by herniation of the brainstem through the foramen magnum in the Arnold–Chiari malformation. Budd–Chiari syndrome is a disorder of hepatic vein occlusion. Vocal cord palsy may present with stridor, dyphonia and aspiration that may lead to pneumonia. Treatment may be conservative or may involve surgery to medialise the vocal cord. Surgery may involve a temporary medialisation by injection, or the implantation of a solid material, as in the Isshiki type I thyroplasty.

62. Answers: TFTTF

Septoplasty is complicated by septal perforation in around 1% of cases, usually due to submucous resection of cartilage in the region of two opposing mucosal tears. Over-resection of septal cartilage can lead to collapse of the supratip region and a saddle-nose deformity. Polly beak deformity describes a dorsal nasal convexity which usually occurs as a complication of rhinoplasty. Anosmia and palatal or dental anaesthesia are recognised complications and are due to neurological injury. Frey syndrome (gustatory sweating) may complicate parotidectomy.

63. The cilia of the nasal mucosa:
    - Have a 9 + 2 microtubular structure
    - Beat at a frequency of approximately 120 Hz
    - Are dysfunctional in Kartagener syndrome
    - May be functionally assessed by the saccharin test
    - May be functionally assessed by nasal brush biopsy

64. The nasolacrimal duct:
    - Drains into the inferior meatus
    - Is approximately 4 cm long
    - Is at risk during septoplasty
    - Is demonstrable on CT scanning
    - Obstruction is more common in females

65. Reinke's oedema:
    - Is also known as dysphonia plica ventricularis
    - Is strongly associated with smoking
    - Voice therapy may be helpful
    - Use of a CO_2 laser is contraindicated
    - Is best managed surgically by stripping the vocal cord

63.   Answers: TFTTT

Motile cilia line the respiratory tract and together with the mucociliary blanket work to keep these areas free from potential pathogens. Motile cilia generally have nine microtubule doublets around the periphery, and a pair of microtubules in the centre, which cross-link to cause beating 10–12 times per second. A variety of disorders of ciliary function have been found in patients with Kartagener syndrome, which is the clinical combination of situs invertus, chronic sinusitis and bronchiectasis. Kartagener syndrome is just one of the broader group of disorders termed primary ciliary dyskinesia. The saccharin test assesses mucociliary clearance, and nasal brush biopsy allows microscopic visualisation of ciliary function.

64.   Answers: TFFTT

The nasolacrimal duct drains tears from the lacrimal sac to the inferior meatus, and is around 12 mm long. It can be injured during surgery to the anterior lateral nasal wall (e.g. sinus surgery), but should not be injured during septoplasty. It is visible on CT scans of the paranasal sinus, and patients may be investigated for epiphora with a CT dacrocystogram. Obstruction is more common in females, for reasons which are unclear.

65.   Answers: FTTFF

Reinke's oedema refers to oedema of the superficial layer of the lamina propria. There is a strong association with smoking, such that the condition is rare in non-smokers. Other associations include voice abuse, hypothyroidism and gastro-oesophageal reflux. Smoking cessation and voice therapy may improve symptoms considerably. If surgery is considered (using either steel or CO_2 laser), aspiration of fluid via a supero-lateral vocal cord incision is preferable, with limited trimming of redundant mucosa. Care should be taken to avoid damaging the underlying vocal cord ligament. Stripping of the vocal cords has no place in current management, and results in a poor voice outcome.

66. Laryngocoele:
    - Has a peak incidence in the third decade of life
    - Is more common in men
    - May be associated with laryngeal carcinoma
    - External laryngocoele is the most common variety
    - Is usually treated with sclerotherapy

67. The frontal sinus:
    - Is usually formed by the age of 3 years
    - Is the origin of Pott disease of the spine
    - Is lined by squamous epithelium
    - Should routinely be explored in the endoscopic treatment of chronic rhinosinusitis
    - Is poorly developed in Crouzon syndrome

68. Hereditary haemorrhagic telangiectasia:
    - Is inherited in an autosomal-dominant fashion
    - Is associated with arteriovenous malformations of the lungs
    - Can be treated using oestrogens
    - Can be treated with a KTP or argon laser
    - Split skin grafts are never effective

66. Answers: FTTFF

A laryngocoele is an abnormal dilatation of the laryngeal saccule. It is more common in men (80%), and has a peak incidence in the fifth and sixth decades of life. It may be classified as internal, external or mixed. Internal laryngocoeles are confined to the larynx and do not penetrate the thyrohyoid membrane. They may extend postero-superiorly into the aryepiglottic fold and false cords, reducing the supraglottic space. External laryngocoeles expand laterally outside the thyrohyoid membrane, exiting in the defect through which the superior laryngeal nerve and vessels pass. Around 50% of laryngocoeles are of the mixed type (the most common presentation), containing features of both. Laryngocoele may in some cases occur secondary to a laryngeal carcinoma. It is suggested that a malignancy may distort the saccule neck and cause a one-way valve effect, increasing intraluminal pressure. Treatment is by endoscopy to identify malignancy, and surgical excision (which may involve removing half of the thyroid cartilage on the side of the lesion in order to provide adequate access to ligate the saccule neck).

67. Answers: FFFFT

The frontal sinus largely develops postnatally. It is radiographically visible at the age of 6 years, but continues to grow on into adulthood. It is continuous with the nasal mucosa, so is lined with pseudostratified columnar ciliated epithelium. Infection can lead to meningitis, brain abscess, orbital cellulitis or osteomyelitis of the frontal bone (so-called Pott's puffy tumour). Sir Percival Pott also described Pott disease of the spine, namely tuberculosis infection of the spine that usually occurs as a consequence of spread from the lungs. The frontal sinus should not be explored routinely during endoscopic sinus surgery, as iatrogenic chronic frontal sinusitis may result. Ethmoidectomy is usually sufficient to allow drainage of the frontal recess. Crouzon syndrome is a disorder characterised by premature fusion of the calvaria; typically frontal sinus and mastoid pneumatisation is reduced.

68. Answers: TTTTF

Hereditary haemorrhagic telangiectasia is an autosomal-dominant condition that is characterised by the presence of mucocutaneous telangiectasia and arteriovenous malformations. Epistaxis and gastrointestinal bleeding are common manifestations of the disease. Oestrogens reduce the haemorrhagic tendency in HHT, and symptoms may worsen following the menopause, due to the oestrogen-deficient state. Argon or KTP laser is a useful treatment for septal lesions. Split skin grafts may be effective, but recurrence is common. Bleeding that is refractory to medical and initial surgical treatments may necessitate a Young's procedure (surgical closure of the nostrils).

69. Septal haematoma:
- Is usually caused by trauma
- Is usually bilateral
- Bleeding occurs in the subperichondrial space
- May lead to a saddle deformity
- Treatment involves intravenous antibiotics and alar pressure

70. Disorders of smell:
- Viral infection may cause anosmia that lasts for more than 2 weeks
- Smoking is a common cause of reduced sense of smell
- Epilepsy is a recognised cause of disordered sense of smell
- The University of Pennsylvania Smell Identification Test (UPSIT) gives a score out of 20
- Ammonia may be used to test the olfactory nerve alone

71. Laryngeal surgery:
- Argon laser is commonly used for the excision of vocal fold lesions
- Surgery is the initial treatment of choice for vocal fold nodules
- Reinke's oedema can be treated surgically
- Surgical treatment of laryngeal papillomatosis is usually curative
- Patients should be advised to whisper following surgery

69.   Answers: TTTTF

Septal haematoma usually occurs following nasal trauma, and is usually bilateral. Blood collects in the plane between the perichondrium of the septal cartilage and the cartilage itself. This results in ischaemia to the cartilage and consequently septal necrosis, which may lead to a saddle deformity. Treatment involves incision and drainage with antibiotic cover.

70.   Answers: TTTFF

Viral infection (e.g. influenza) may cause prolonged anosmia, and spontaneous return of the sense of smell is recognised even up to 2 years after infection. Exposure to cigarette smoke may cause damage to the olfactory epithelium, impairing the sense of smell. Temporal lobe epilepsy may cause olfactory hallucinations. The UPSIT score involves testing with 40 microencapsulated odours, and gives a score out of 40 (patients with anosmia score around 10 out of 40). Ammonia causes stimulation of the trigeminal nerve and therefore cannot be used to test the olfactory nerve alone.

71.   Answers: FFTFF

CO_2 laser is more commonly used for the excision of vocal fold lesions, as it allows precision microsurgery with a relatively bloodless field. It is invisible to the naked eye, and therefore a low-power helium–neon laser is used coaxially as a sighting beam. Argon laser is more commonly used in ophthalmic surgery. Reinke's oedema may be managed surgically if there is no improvement as a result of conservative and medical measures. Laryngeal papillomatosis is associated with frequent recurrences, and surgery is rarely curative. Recently, intralesional antiviral therapy (e.g. cidofovir) has been used at the time of surgery to try to reduce the frequency of recurrences. Whispering may be associated with greater vocal fold trauma than normal speech, and therefore should be avoided following laryngeal surgery.

72. The recurrent laryngeal nerve:
    • Is in close proximity to the superior thyroid artery
    • Supplies the cricothyroid muscle
    • Supplies sensation to the sub-glottic larynx
    • The left recurrent laryngeal nerve loops under the arch of the aorta
    • Bilateral injury may require tracheostomy

73. Epistaxis:
    • The anterior nasal septum is the most common site of bleeding
    • A drop in blood pressure is an early sign of compromise
    • Active epistaxis should be treated by supratip pressure with the patient lying supine
    • Nasal tampons should be used after bleeding has stopped, to prevent further bleeding
    • Antibiotic cover should be used with all nasal packing

72. Answers: FFTTT

The recurrent laryngeal nerve supplies motor innervation to all of the muscles of the larynx except the cricothyroid (which is supplied by the superior laryngeal nerve). It also supplies sensory innervation to the laryngeal mucosa below the vocal cords. It is closely related to the inferior thyroid artery. The left recurrent laryngeal nerve loops under the aortic arch, whereas the right recurrent laryngeal nerve loops under the subclavian artery. Recurrent laryngeal nerve injury may lead to ipsilateral vocal fold palsy. If there is bilateral vocal cord palsy, tracheostomy may be required to overcome airway obstruction.

73. Answers: TFFFF

The most common site of epistaxis is Little's area on the antero-inferior nasal septum. Kiesselbach's plexus overlies this area, representing an anastamosis of several arterial branches from the internal and external carotid arteries. A drop in blood pressure is a late sign of cardiovascular compromise. An increase in pulse and a rise in respiratory rate are earlier indicators. In most cases of epistaxis, alar pressure (over Little's area) with the patient sitting upright and leaning forward (to limit the amount of blood swallowed by the patient) is a good first intervention. Nasal tamponade can be used if this fails to achieve haemostasis, but this may be counter-productive if haemostasis has been achieved, as trauma due to insertion of nasal tampons may cause further bleeding. There are no agreed guidelines for the use of antibiotics with nasal packing, but many ENT surgeons advocate the use of antibiotic cover if packs are left *in situ* for more than 48 hours.

Head and neck

74. Causes of facial palsy include:
  - Parotid neoplasm
  - Charcot–Marie–Tooth disease
  - Tick bites
  - Stapedotomy
  - Otitis media

75. Indications for tonsillectomy include:
  - Recurrent quinsy
  - Debulking of Ann Arbor stage 3 lymphoma
  - Adult obstructive sleep apnoea
  - Acute tonsillitis
  - Cogan syndrome

76. Craniofacial malformations that can affect the paediatric airway include:
  - Crouzon syndrome
  - Maxillary hyperostosis
  - Pfeiffer syndrome
  - Fragile X syndrome
  - Pierre Robin sequence

74.   Answers: TFTTT

There are many causes of facial palsy. Parotid malignancies must be ruled out, especially when a palsy fails to recover. Lyme disease transmitted by tick bites is another cause. Iatrogenic facial palsy may occur following middle ear or parotid surgery, and occasionally following stapedotomy (either immediately following surgery or as a delayed presentation). Suppurative otitis media can sometimes cause facial palsy, especially if the facial nerve is dehiscent in the middle ear. Charcot–Marie–Tooth disease refers to a hereditary sensory and motor neuropathy that affects the peripheral nerves.

75.   Answers: TFTTF

Common indications for tonsillectomy are recurrent infections, including quinsy. However, occasionally a 'hot tonsillectomy' may be indicated for an acute infection that does not respond to usual therapy. Tonsillectomy is also indicated for diagnostic purposes when there is a suspicion of malignancy such as lymphoma or squamous-cell carcinoma. Tonsillectomy may occasionally be used to debulk disease in squamous-cell carcinoma, but lymphoma is treated with chemotherapy or radiotherapy. Tonsillectomy can also be used to treat paediatric and occasionally adult obstructive sleep apnoea. Cogan syndrome is a rare autoimmune disorder that predominantly affects the eye and inner ear. It is unrelated to the tonsils.

76.   Answers: TFTFT

Crouzon and Pfeiffer syndromes are caused by genetic mutations in fibroblast-growth-factor receptors, which lead to premature fusion of the calvaria and poor midface development. The latter can lead to a reduced nasopharyngeal airway. Pierre Robin sequence is caused by mandibular hypoplasia, which leads to inadequate anatomical space for tongue development, and consequent cleft palate due to physical obstruction to the fusion of the palatal shelves. The tongue base may impinge upon the airway. Maxillary hyperostosis and fragile X syndrome do not compromise the airway.

77. Orbital cellulitis:
- Often arises from maxillary sinusitis in children
- Is a cause of proptosis
- May be caused by *Haemophilus influenzae*
- Can cause meningitis
- May require endoscopic decompression

78. Cleft palate:
- Is a heritable disorder
- May be diagnosed *in utero*
- Is associated with Stickler syndrome
- Is associated with bifid uvula
- Has a higher incidence in the African population

79. A 5-year-old child presents with a midline cystic swelling 1 cm below the hyoid bone:
- Movement with tongue protrusion is suggestive of a thyroglossal cyst
- Ultrasound is a useful investigation
- This is best treated by incision and drainage
- This often resolves spontaneously
- The cyst is usually associated with a lingual thyroid

77. Answers: FTTTT

Orbital cellulitis can arise from spread of infection from the ethmoid sinuses (rarely from the maxillary sinuses), from orbital injury or from bacteraemia. When spread from the ethmoid sinuses, respiratory pathogens are often responsible, such as streptococci or *Haemophilus influenzae*. The cardinal signs are proptosis and ophthalmoplegia. Treatment must be prompt to prevent complications of visual loss or further spread of infection (e.g. meningitis). If antibiotics are ineffective, surgical drainage or decompression is indicated, especially if an orbital abscess develops. This may be approached externally, but endoscopic techniques may also be used.

78. Answers: TTTTF

Cleft palate results from failure of fusion of the palatal shelves. It is a heritable disorder, with many genes thought to be involved, but no racial predilection has been noted. It can be diagnosed *in utero* by ultrasound scanning. Hundreds of syndromes are associated with cleft palate, and Stickler syndrome (a collagen disorder) is one of them. A bifid uvula can be a sign of submucous cleft palate.

79. Answers: TTFFF

Movement with tongue protrusion is the classical sign of a thyroglossal cyst, due to attachment to the hyoid bone (but this is not always demonstrable). Ultrasound is a useful investigation because it confirms no associated (rare) embryological failure of thyroid gland development. Incision and drainage are undesirable if a cyst is infected, due to the risk of scarring and sinus formation. Antibiotic therapy and aspiration of the cyst are preferable. Often the cyst is persistent, and when inflammation has resolved, excision by Sistrunk's procedure is the operation of choice.

80. The following are branches of the facial nerve:
- Buccal
- Frontal
- Chorda tympani
- Zygomatic
- Posterior auricular nerve

81. Lymphatic malformation (cystic hygroma):
- Most commonly affects the anterior triangle of the neck
- Is more common in females
- May present with a failure to thrive
- Can cause upper airway obstruction
- May be treated with surgery or laser

82. The lateral pterygoid muscle:
- Is attached to the medial surface of the lateral pterygoid plate
- Is attached to the intra-articular disc of the TMJ
- Retracts the mandible
- Is supplied by the maxillary branch of the trigeminal nerve
- Is composed of smooth muscle

80. Answers: TFTTT

The facial nerve contains somatic sensory, taste, general and visceral motor fibres. The chorda tympani joins the lingual branch of the mandibular division of the trigeminal nerve to supply taste to the anterior two-thirds of the tongue. After it exits the stylomastoid foramen, the facial nerve gives off branches to the posterior belly digastric muscle and stylohyoid, and the posterior auricular nerve. The main trunk of the nerve usually divides into anterior (superior) and posterior (inferior) divisions within the parotid gland. The anterior (superior) division gives off temporal and zygomatic branches. The posterior (inferior) division gives rise to the buccal, mandibular and cervical branches.

81. Answers: FFTTT

Lymphatic malformation most commonly affects the posterior triangle of the neck. The sex distribution is equal. Signs and symptoms vary according to the location of the lesion. Patients may present with significant neck swelling, failure to thrive, or even airway obstruction. A temporary tracheostomy may be required. Treatment options include surgical excision, laser excision or sclerotherapy.

82. Answers: FTFFF

The lower head of the lateral pterygoid muscle is attached to the lateral surface of the lateral pterygoid plate. It inserts into the capsule of the TMJ and is attached to the intra-articular disc of the TMJ. It acts to protrude the mandible and open the mouth. It is supplied by the anterior division of the mandibular nerve (V) and is composed of striated muscle.

83. The temporo-mandibular joint (TMJ):
    • Is a synovial joint
    • Its articular surfaces are lined by fibrous cartilage
    • Has an anterior and posterior compartment
    • Forward dislocation is more common
    • Dislocation is more common when the masseteric muscles are relaxed

84. Branches of the external carotid artery include:
    • Lingual artery
    • Inferior thyroid artery
    • Ascending cervical artery
    • Facial artery
    • Superficial temporal artery

85. Parotid pleomorphic adenoma:
    • Is more common in men
    • Is usually mobile on palpation
    • Commonly results in a facial nerve palsy
    • Can often be diagnosed by fine-needle aspiration cytology
    • Radiotherapy is the treatment of choice

83. Answers: TTFTT

The TMJ is a synovial joint with articular surfaces lined by fibro-cartilage. The TMJ has upper and lower compartments, which are separated by the intra-articular disc. Dislocation is most commonly anterior, with the mandibular head passing forward over the articular tubercle. Masseteric tone acts to prevent anterior dislocation, so muscle relaxants that are given during general anaesthesia leave the TMJ at risk of dislocation during manipulation. It is important to remember this when inserting the Boyle–Davis gag for a tonsillectomy.

84. Answers: TFFTT

The major branches of the external carotid artery include the superior thyroid, ascending pharyngeal, lingual, facial, occipital, posterior auricular, maxillary and superficial temporal branches. The inferior thyroid artery arises from the thyrocervical trunk of the subclavian artery.

85. Answers: FTFTF

Pleomorphic adenomas are more common in women. They are highly mobile, and although they may be intimately related to the facial nerve, invasion resulting in facial nerve palsy does not occur. Fine-needle aspiration cytology may identify pleomorphic adenoma. Surgery in the form of parotidectomy is the treatment of choice.

86. Early signs of perforation following oesophagoscopy include:
- Tachycardia
- Chest pain
- Dysphagia
- Hypotension
- Low urine output

87. The anterior triangle of the neck:
- Is bordered anteriorly by the anterior border of sternocleido-mastoid
- Contains the strap muscles of the neck
- Includes the carotid and digastric triangles
- Contains the accessory nerve
- Contains the internal jugular vein

88. The mandibular division of the trigeminal nerve:
- Divides into anterior and posterior divisions
- Is sensory and motor
- Leaves the skull base through the foramen rotundum
- Supplies the masseter muscle
- Gives off a lingual branch

86. Answers: TTFTF

Tachycardia, chest pain and hypotension are early signs of oesophageal perforation. Pyrexia and tachypnoea post-operatively are also red flags. Post-operative instructions should especially highlight the need to contact the ENT surgeon on call if abnormalities in these parameters develop.

87. Answers: FTTFT

The anterior triangle of the neck is bordered by the inferior border of the mandible, the anterior border of the sternocleidomastoid and the midline of the neck. It contains all of the strap muscles of the neck, except the inferior belly of omohyoid. It can be divided into carotid, digastric and submental triangles. Both anterior jugular veins and the internal jugular vein are contained in the anterior triangle. The accessory nerve runs within the posterior triangle.

88. Answers: TTFTT

The mandibular division of the trigeminal nerve leaves the skull base through the foramen ovale. The anterior division gives motor branches to the temporalis, lateral pterygoid and masseter muscles, and a small sensory buccal branch. The posterior division gives rise to auriculotemporal, lingual and inferior alveolar branches.

89. The posterior triangle of the neck:
- The floor is formed from prevertebral fascia
- Is bordered anteriorly by the posterior border of sternocleido-mastoid
- Contains branches of the cervical plexus
- Contains the vagus nerve
- Is the most common site of lymphatic malformation (cystic hygroma)

90. Warthin's tumour (salivary gland adenolymphoma):
- Is more common in young women
- Is associated with cigarette smoking
- Recurrence is common
- May be adequately treated with radiotherapy
- Is composed largely of squamous epithelium

91. Complications of facial palsy:
- Bell's palsy results in permanent facial weakness in 50% of cases
- Ramsay Hunt syndrome results in complete recovery of facial function in 90% of cases
- Gustatory sweating is a recognised complication
- Corneal abrasion is a recognised complication
- Prednisolone reduces the risk of permanent facial weakness in Bell's palsy

89. Answers: TTTFT

The posterior triangle is bordered by the posterior border of the sterno-cleidomastoid, the anterior border of the trapezius and the middle third of the clavicle. The roof is formed from the investing layer of deep fascia and the floor consists of prevertebral fascia. The accessory nerve, and branches of the cervical and brachial plexus are found within the posterior triangle.

90. Answers: FTFFF

Warthin's tumour is a benign tumour of the salivary gland that is more common in elderly men. There is a strong association with cigarette smoking. Following surgical excision, recurrence is rare, and radiotherapy has no role. Warthin's tumour may be bilateral in around 10% of cases, but rarely synchronously.

91. Answers: FFFTT

Bell's palsy is idiopathic facial nerve palsy, and is a diagnosis of exclusion. It is associated with complete recovery in about 85% of cases, and early treatment with steroids increases the likelihood of recovery. Ramsay Hunt syndrome has a worse prognosis, with complete recovery rates of less than 50%. If there is incomplete eye closure as a result of facial palsy, there is a risk of corneal abrasions and the patient should use aqueous tears and tape the affected eye shut at night. Gustatory sweating (Frey syndrome) occurs following parotid surgery.

92. Hypopharyngeal carcinoma:
    • Has a poor prognosis
    • Is uncommon and usually affects younger patients
    • There is a very strong association with smoking
    • The piriform fossa is the most commonly involved site
    • Post-cricoid carcinoma is associated with Paterson–Brown-Kelly syndrome

93. Oral cavity carcinoma:
    • Most commonly affects the lateral border of the tongue and the floor of the mouth
    • Is associated with smoking and alcohol
    • MRI scan is useful for assessing bony invasion
    • A T3 tumour is greater than 4 cm in its greatest dimension
    • Following tumour excision, patients should be followed up yearly

94. The submandibular gland:
    • Produces around 30% of saliva in the adult
    • Has a superficial and deep lobe
    • The lingual nerve crosses the submandibular duct superiorly from medial to lateral
    • The facial artery runs superficial to the gland
    • Must be excised by an incision 1 cm below the mandible to avoid nerve injury

92.   Answers: TFFTT

The hypopharynx includes the post-cricoid region, the piriform fossa and posterior pharyngeal wall. Tumours in this region are usually squamous-cell carcinomas and generally present in elderly men. The association of smoking and alcohol with hypopharyngeal carcinoma is not as strong as that with laryngeal carcinoma. Hypopharyngeal tumours most commonly affect the piriform fossa. Paterson–Brown-Kelly syndrome refers to the presence of iron-deficiency anaemia and a post-cricoid web. This is associated with an increased risk of post-cricoid carcinoma.

93.   Answers: TTFTF

The lateral border of the tongue and the floor of the mouth are the most common sites of carcinoma of the oral cavity. There is a strong association with smoking, alcohol and betel nut chewing. CT imaging is more useful for assessing bony invasion than MRI. A T2 tumour is more than 2 cm but less than 4 cm in its greatest dimension. A T3 tumour is larger than 4 cm. Any tumour with extension to bone, muscle or skin is defined as T4. The highest risk of recurrence in within the first year, so initial follow-up after treatment should be every few weeks.

94.   Answers: FTFFF

The submandibular gland produces around 70% of saliva volume. It is composed of a superficial lobe, which communicates with a smaller deep lobe around the posterior border of the mylohyoid muscle. The blood supply is from the lingual and facial arteries. The facial artery runs deep to the gland. The lingual nerve runs lateral to the submandibular duct, and then crosses it running inferiorly and then medial to it. The incision for submandibular gland excision is at least two finger-breadths (of the patient) below the mandible (around 2.5 cm in the adult male) to avoid the marginal mandibular branch of the facial nerve.

95. The tongue:
- Receives its blood supply from branches of the external carotid artery
- The chorda tympani supplies sympathetic fibres
- The glossopharyngeal nerve supplies taste and sensation to the posterior third
- The hypoglossal nerve is the motor supply to all the muscles of the tongue
- Deviates to the left with a left hypoglossal nerve palsy

96. Papillary adenocarcinoma of the thyroid:
- Is the most common malignant thyroid tumour
- Usually presents as a single thyroid nodule
- Lymph node spread is very rare
- Tumours smaller than 3 cm may be treated with hemi-thyroidectomy alone
- TSH suppression below normal levels is a component of treatment following surgery

97. Follicular adenocarcinoma of the thyroid:
- Is more common in young women
- Accounts for around 10% of all thyroid malignancies
- Diagnosis can be confirmed by fine-needle aspiration cytology
- May spread via the bloodstream
- Can often be treated with levothyroxine alone

95.   Answers: TFTFT

The tongue receives its blood supply from lingual branches of the external carotid artery. The anterior two-thirds of the tongue receive sensory innervation from the lingual nerve, and taste fibres from the chorda tympani. The posterior third receives sensory and taste innervation from the glossopharyngeal nerve. The hypoglossal nerve supplies the intrinsic and extrinsic muscles of the tongue except for the palatoglossus (which is supplied by the pharyngeal plexus).

96.   Answers: TTFFT

Papillary adenocarcinoma is the most common thyroid malignancy, accounting for around 80% of cases. It is more common in women, and usually presents as a solitary nodule. Spread to lymph nodes is present in around 50% of cases, but this does not adversely affect the prognosis. Tumours greater than 1 cm in diameter are defined as high risk under the British Thyroid Association guidelines, and total thyroidectomy is recommended. Lifelong suppression of TSH is mandatory, as the tumours are hormone sensitive.

97.   Answers: FTFTF

Follicular carcinoma is seen in an older age group than papillary carcinoma, with a peak incidence between 40 and 60 years of age. It is not possible to differentiate between follicular adenoma and adenocarcinoma on the basis of fine-needle aspiration cytology. Follicular carcinoma may spread by the haematogenous route, giving rise to pulmonary or bony metastases. Treatment involves hemithyroidectomy or total thyroidectomy and radioiodine treatment.

98. Parotid surgery:
- Pleomorphic adenomas are best treated by enucleation of the tumour
- A facial nerve stimulator may be used to assist the surgeon
- Numbness of the ear lobe is a recognised complication
- Facial nerve weakness following surgery is permanent in the majority of cases
- Use of a drain is contraindicated

99. Anaplastic carcinoma of the thyroid:
- Most commonly occurs in elderly women
- Shows rapid invasion of local structures
- Commonly occurs in the setting of a pre-existing goitre
- Five-year survival is around 50%
- Surgery is curative in most cases

100. Complications of tracheostomy include:
- Pneumothorax
- Erosion of the external carotid artery
- Permanent fistula
- Pneumonia
- Guillain–Barré syndrome

98.   Answers: FTTFF

Pleomorphic adenoma is the most common benign salivary neoplasm. Recurrence may occur if the capsule is ruptured during removal. Depending upon the site of the tumour, obtaining as wide a margin as possible is preferred (e.g. by superficial parotidectomy). Injury to the great auricular nerve may give rise to numbness of the earlobe. Facial nerve weakness post-operatively is usually due to a neuropraxia, which resolves in the majority of cases. Drains are not contraindicated, but should be positioned carefully to avoid direct suction on branches of the facial nerve.

99.   Answers: TTTFF

Anaplastic carcinoma is an aggressive locally invasive cancer that is associated with an extremely poor prognosis. It may occur in the setting of a long-standing multinodular goitre. Histologically it may be difficult to differentiate anaplastic carcinoma from lymphoma. Treatment is often palliative, in the form of radiotherapy with or without surgery. Tracheostomy may be required to relieve distressing airway obstruction.

100.   Answers: TFTTF

Significant haemorrhage occurs following around 5% of tracheostomies. Massive haemorrhage can occur as a result of erosion of the innominate artery or sometimes the right common carotid artery. The external carotid artery begins above the trachea and so is not at risk. Pneumothorax complicates tracheostomy in around 2% of adult cases, but is more common in children. As with endotracheal intubation, pneumonia may occur because regions of significant mucosal immune function are bypassed. Occasionally a permanent fistula may result from tracheostomy; the incidence is related to the duration of intubation. Other complications include infection, tube obstruction, tracheal granulation and tracheo-oesophageal fistula. Guillain–Barré syndrome is a demyelinating autoimmune peripheral neuropathy that can lead to respiratory failure and the need for long-term ventilatory support, including tracheostomy. However, it is not a complication of tracheostomy.

101. The following are indications for tracheostomy:
- Nasopharyngeal carcinoma
- Obstructive sleep apnoea
- Bilateral vocal cord palsy
- Facial trauma
- Epiglottitis

102. The following are risk factors for thyroid cancer:
- Female sex
- Family history
- Previous radiotherapy to the neck
- Multiple endocrine neoplasia type 2
- Branchial cyst

103. Post-operative chylous fistula:
- Occurs more commonly on the left side
- Is a complication of supraomohyoid neck dissection
- May require total parenteral nutrition as part of treatment
- Can lead to hypoproteinaemia
- Occurs in 20% of neck dissections

101. Answers: FTTTT

There are many indications for tracheostomy. The most common reason is to minimise the risk of subglottic stenosis from prolonged endo-tracheal intubation. Tracheostomy is also commonly used to overcome obstructions above the proximal trachea, whether due to tumours impinging upon the larynx, injuries such as displaced facial fractures, bilateral vocal cord palsy, infections such as epiglottitis, or even severe obstructive sleep apnoea. Nasopharyngeal carcinoma compromises the nasal airway but not the oral airway, and it is very unlikely that there will be a need for tracheostomy. Occasionally tracheostomy is also indicated to reduce physiological dead space to improve gaseous exchange, or to permit pulmonary toilet.

102. Answers: TTTTF

Thyroid carcinoma is around three times more frequent in females than in males. External beam radiotherapy is a risk factor in aetiology. Multiple endocrine neoplasia types 2A and 2B are genetic defects that lead to an increased risk of medullary carcinoma in affected families. However, the risk of papillary and follicular carcinoma is also increased in some families, through unidentified mechanisms. Branchial cyst is not a risk factor for thyroid cancer, although occasionally metastatic thyroid carcinoma may be mistaken for a branchial cyst.

103. Answers: TFTTF

Chylous fistula results from damage to lymphatic structures in the lower neck, usually the thoracic duct close to where it enters the subclavian vein on the left. A neck dissection that does not include the lower neck (e.g. supraomohyoid) does not risk causing a chylous fistula. Because chyle contains 20–30 g/L of protein, hypoproteinaemia is a risk, as is hyponatraemia, acidosis and hypocalcaemia. Treatment is conservative for low-volume leaks, and may include pressure dressing and total parenteral nutrition. Surgery is indicated for high-volume leaks or those that fail conservative management. Chylous fistula occurs in around 2% of neck dissections.

104. Facial haemangiomas:
- Are more common in males
- Can be treated conservatively in the majority of cases
- Are associated with neurofibromatosis type 1
- Are responsive to oral corticosteroids
- Are associated with subglottic haemangioma

105. Complications of endotracheal intubation include:
- Subglottic stenosis
- Anterior glottic web
- Vocal process granuloma
- Vocal cord paralysis
- Thyroid storm

106. Complications of radiotherapy to the head and neck include:
- Xerostomia
- Necrosis of bone
- Hepatic dysfunction
- Cataract formation
- Thyroid cancer

104. Answers: FTFTT

Facial haemangiomas are common vascular malformations that are most often seen in female Caucasian infants. There is an association with haemangiomas elsewhere, and the development of stridor in an infant with facial haemangioma may indicate a subglottic haemangioma. Almost all haemangiomas can be treated conservatively, as they will regress, but intervention may be necessary if they are interfering with visual function or breathing. In the proliferative phase they respond to systemic or sometimes intralesional steroids. Laser surgical excision is rarely required. Skin lesions in neurofibromatosis type 1 include neurofibromas, café au lait spots and freckling of the groin or axilla, but not haemangiomas.

105. Answers: TFTTF

Endotracheal intubation can cause a variety of injuries to the larynx or trachea. Vocal process granulomas occur in an estimated 1 in 10 000 intubations, and are usually treated conservatively. Vocal cord paralysis may rarely occur due to a high-pressure cuff causing injury to the anterior division of the inferior (recurrent) laryngeal nerve. Anterior glottic web is a congenital failure of full canalisation of the larynx. Thyroid storm is an acute exacerbation of hyperthyroidism caused by physiological stress, including surgery. However, endotracheal intubation per se is not the cause.

106. Answers: TTFTT

Radiotherapy to the head and neck will cause acute mucositis in the majority of patients, as well as xerostomia (dry mouth). Whereas the mucositis will settle, the xerostomia may be chronic due to degeneration and fibrosis in the acini of the salivary glands. Osteoradionecrosis typically affects the mandible and is due to the death of osteocytes. It may either occur spontaneously or be triggered by trauma such as dental extraction. The eyes and spinal cord are generally spared from the radiotherapy field. However, in for example locally invasive sinonasal malignancy, the eye may be exposed to radiation which can lead to later problems such as cataract formation or corneal ulceration. The risk of thyroid cancer is increased in individuals with a history of previous radiotherapy to the neck. Chemotherapy can cause hepatic dysfunction, but there is no effect from radiotherapy if it does not include the liver in the irradiated field.

107. The following are branches of the trigeminal (V) nerve:
- Supraorbital nerve
- Lingual nerve
- Nasopalatine nerve
- Nerve to mylohyoid
- Nerve to stapedius

108. Tracheomalacia:
- Can be caused by prolonged endotracheal intubation
- May be associated with maldevelopment of branchial arch arteries
- Is graded by the Cotton classification
- May be diagnosed by ultrasound
- Can be treated with continuous positive airway pressure (CPAP)

109. Complications of bilateral radical neck dissection include:
- Shoulder pain
- Raised intracranial pressure
- Carotid artery rupture
- Hypothyroidism
- Dysphonia

107. Answers: TTTTF

The trigeminal nerve has three sensory divisions – ophthalmic (V1), maxillary (V2) and mandibular (V3) – which together supply general sensation to the face, oral cavity and nasal cavity, and relay post-ganglionic parasympathetic fibres to their target organ. In addition, the mandibular division carries motor fibres to the muscles of mastication. The supraorbital nerve is a division of V1, the nasopalatine nerve is a division of V2 and the lingual nerve and the nerve to mylohyoid are divisions of V3. The nerve to the stapedius is a branch of the facial (VII) nerve.

108. Answers: TTFFT

Tracheomalacia is a weakness of the tracheal wall. It may be intrinsic or congenital (type 1), caused by external compression (typically from a vascular ring resulting from branchial arch artery anomalies) (type 2), or caused by prolonged intubation or chronic tracheitis (type 3). Treatment may be conservative, including the use of positive pressure to stent open the collapsing airway. Surgical treatment for resistant cases includes tracheostomy, aortopexy and tracheal stents. The Cotton classification is used for subglottic stenosis. Ultrasound has no place in diagnosis. Cinefluoroscopy, dynamic CT or endoscopic visualisation are the usual means of making a diagnosis.

109. Answers: TTTFT

Several structures are at risk in a radical neck dissection, including the vagus nerve, injury to which will lead to dysphonia due to vocal cord paralysis. In a bilateral radical neck dissection, both internal jugular veins will be tied off, which will raise the intracranial pressure by up to 40 mmHg. In addition, both accessory nerves will be sacrificed, which leads to shoulder pain. Carotid artery rupture can occur due to wound breakdown, particularly in the previously irradiated neck. It occurs in around 3% of neck dissections and is usually fatal. Thyroid tissue is not removed in a radical neck dissection, so hypothyroidism would not be expected.

110. Pharyngeal pouch (Zenker's diverticulum):
   • Is more common in men
   • Arises between the middle and inferior constrictor muscles
   • Usually presents as a palpable mass in the anterior triangle of the neck
   • May initially be treated with oral hyoscine
   • Is best imaged with MRI

111. Sjögren syndrome:
   • Primary Sjögren syndrome may be caused by rheumatoid arthritis
   • It affects the salivary glands in around 10% of cases
   • Schirmer test may be performed in the outpatient setting
   • Tru-cut biopsy is the diagnostic test of choice
   • Serum ANCA is useful for diagnosis

112. The pterygopalatine fossa:
   • Communicates with the orbit
   • Contains the maxillary artery
   • Contains the otic ganglion
   • Is a common site for juvenile angiofibroma
   • Is immediately lateral to the anterior ethmoid sinus

110. Answers: TFFFF

Pharyngeal pouch is most common in the elderly and in men. It is a herniation of the oesophageal mucosa between the thyropharyngeus and cricopharyngeus parts of the inferior constrictor muscle, and is thought to arise due to incoordinated muscle activity in this region. It usually presents with symptoms of dysphagia, delayed regurgitation of food, aspiration, halitosis or dysphonia. It is rare for there to be a palpable mass. The diagnosis is made by barium swallow. No medical treatment has been shown to work. Surgical treatment usually involves endoscopic stapling and division of the party wall between the pouch and the adjacent oesophagus.

111. Answers: FFTFF

Sjögren syndrome is an autoimmune disease that is characterised by the symptoms of dry mouth and decreased tear production. Primary Sjögren syndrome refers to xerostomia and xerophthalmia with no other connective tissue disease. Secondary Sjögren syndrome refers to an association with another connective tissue disease (e.g. rheumatoid arthritis). The salivary glands are involved in around 40% of cases. Schirmer test involves measuring the length of filter paper that is moistened by tears when placed inside the lower eyelid for 5 minutes. Patients with Sjögren syndrome moisten a significantly shorter length of filter paper, due to decreased tear production. Sjögren syndrome is associated with the presence of anti-Ro (SS-A) and anti-La (SS-B) antibodies. Serum ANCA is not useful for diagnosis.

112. Answers: TTFTF

The pterygopalatine fossa is an area between the maxillary antrum (anteriorly), the greater wing of the sphenoid (posteriorly) and the palatine bone (medially). It is lateral to the nasopharynx. It communicates with the orbit through the inferior orbital fissure, and contains the third part of the maxillary artery and the pterygopalatine ganglion (the otic ganglion is in the infratemporal fossa). Juvenile angiofibroma arises near the sphenopalatine foramen in adolescent males, and is a dumbbell-shaped lesion that extends medially into the nasopharynx (where it presents with epistaxis) and laterally into the pterygopalatine fossa.

113. Oral leucoplakia:
     • Is associated with tobacco use
     • Is frequently painful
     • May become malignant
     • Usually requires biopsy for definitive diagnosis
     • Is more common in women

114. The hypoglossal nerve:
     • Exits the skull through the jugular foramen
     • Supplies the styloglossus muscle
     • Passes between the internal and external carotid artery
     • Relays C3 nerve fibres
     • Is at risk in submandibular gland excision

115. Thyroid eye disease:
     • Is a consequence of Graves disease
     • Is more common in women
     • May cause optic neuropathy
     • Is often controlled with carbimazole
     • May be decompressed endoscopically

113. Answers: TFTTF

Oral leucoplakia is an asymptomatic white patch on the oral mucosa that cannot be rubbed off. It occurs more frequently in men, and typically in people aged 40–70 years. Although the cause is uncertain, there is a link with tobacco smoking. It is regarded as pre-malignant, and 10% may at some stage develop malignant features. Biopsy is therefore necessary with subsequent regular close monitoring and repeat biopsy if necessary.

114. Answers: FTFFT

The hypoglossal nerve is the twelfth cranial nerve. It arises from the hypoglossal nucleus in the medulla and exits the cranium through the hypoglossal canal. It then runs lateral to the internal carotid artery, between this and the internal jugular vein. It is joined by C1 fibres of the descendens hypoglossi, which are destined for the infrahyoid muscles of the neck (sternothyroid, thyrohyoid, omohyoid and geniohyoid). The hypoglossal nerve itself supplies all of the intrinsic and extrinsic muscles of the tongue except the palatoglossus (which is supplied by the pharyngeal plexus). The nerve is at risk during neck dissection or submandibular gland excision.

115. Answers: TTTFT

Thyroid eye disease occurs in patients with Graves disease. This disease is caused by an autoimmune antibody to the TSH receptor which leads to hyperthyroidism. It is thought that the same antibodies cross-react with antigens in the retro-orbital space to cause eye disease. The disease is more common in women, although the most severe form of the disease occurs in men. There is lymphocytic infiltration of the retro-orbital space, activation of fibroblasts and oedema of the extra-ocular muscles. Because the orbit is an enclosed space, such swelling causes proptosis of the globe and in some cases the pressure may also cause optic neuropathy. The latter requires urgent treatment. The disease tends to be self-limiting, but severe cases may require systemic steroid treatment or even radiotherapy, although neither of these provides long-term benefit. Treatment of the hyperthyroidism (e.g. with carbimazole) has little or no effect upon eye disease. In refractory cases, surgical decompression is warranted. Trans-orbital, trans-antral or endoscopic sinus approaches may be used to remove the inferior and medial orbital walls. In very rare severe cases a four-wall decompression can be achieved via a neurosurgical approach.

116. The glossopharyngeal nerve:
- Has both sensory and motor branches
- Passes through the foramen rotundum
- Has the greater petrosal nerve as a branch
- Supplies the hyoglossus muscle
- Supplies taste sensation to the posterior third of the tongue

117. The following are contents of the infratemporal fossa:
- Otic ganglion
- Chorda tympani
- Medial pterygoid
- Buccinator
- Maxillary artery

118. Neck injuries:
- Are more common in men
- If penetrating are usually due to a road traffic accident
- Should be immediately explored in the emergency department if platysma is breached
- May cause Brown–Sequard syndrome
- Are a recognised indication for tracheostomy

116. Answers: TFFFT

The glossopharyngeal nerve contains somatic sensory and visceral motor fibres. The nerve passes anterolaterally into the anterior compartment of the jugular foramen. The lesser petrosal nerve is formed from the tympanic branch of the glossopharyngeal nerve which mingles with parasympathetic fibres from the facial nerve. The greater petrosal nerve is derived from the facial nerve and contains no contributions from the glossopharyngeal nerve. The glossopharyngeal nerve supplies the stylopharyngeus muscle. All of the tongue muscles except the palatoglossus (which is supplied by the pharyngeal plexus) are supplied by the hypoglossal nerve. The glossopharyngeal nerve supplies both taste and somatic sensation to the posterior third of the tongue.

117. Answers: TTTFT

The infratemporal fossa lies below and medial to the zygomatic arch. It contains both medial and lateral pterygoids, the lower part of temporalis, the maxillary artery and the pterygoid venous plexus. Nerves that pass within the infratemporal fossa include branches of the mandibular nerve and the chorda tympani. The otic ganglion is a parasympathetic ganglion located immediately below the foramen rotundum in the infratemporal fossa.

118. Answers: TFFTT

Neck injuries may be classified as penetrating or blunt. Penetrating injuries are usually due to stab or gunshot wounds. Blunt injuries are usually due to road traffic accidents or attempted hanging/strangulation. Neck injuries are more common in men. A variety of structures in the neck may be damaged. If the larynx or other parts of the airway are severely disrupted, there may be a need for intubation or even tracheostomy. Penetrating injury deep to platysma carries a 50% risk of major vessel damage, and such wounds should not be explored in the emergency department, but in the operating theatre. Some cases of penetrating neck injury may be treated with observation rather than surgical exploration, but this is an area of contention. Brown–Sequard syndrome is a loss of sensation and motor function due to spinal cord hemitransection.

119. The thyroid gland:
- Develops from the fourth and fifth pharyngeal pouches
- Secretes thyroglobulin
- Has an increased risk of malignancy in smokers
- Receives its blood supply from the subclavian and external carotid arteries
- Is involved in calcium homeostasis

120. Salivary calculi:
- Occur most frequently in the parotid gland
- Are usually radio-opaque
- May be removed through an oral incision
- May be removed endoscopically
- Are a cause of Ludwig's angina

121. Barrett's oesophagus:
- Refers to metaplasia of squamous cells of the upper oesophagus
- Predominantly affects females
- Is a complication of gastro-oesophageal reflux disease
- Is a strong risk factor for squamous-cell carcinoma of the oesophagus
- The treatment of choice is steroid therapy

119. Answers: FTFTT

The thyroid gland develops from the foramen caecum of the tongue from elements derived from the third and fourth pharyngeal pouches. The follicular cells of the thyroid secrete thyroglobulin and thyroid hormones (T3 and T4), whereas the parafollicular C cells secrete calcitonin, which lowers serum calcium levels. The blood supply is from the inferior thyroid artery, a branch of the thyrocervical trunk (subclavian artery) and the superior thyroid artery (external carotid artery). The risk of thyroid malignancy in smokers is actually less than that in non-smokers.

120. Answers: FTTTT

Around 80% of salivary calculi occur in the submandibular gland, and almost all of the remainder occur in the parotid. Salivary calculi are composed of a variety of constituents, but usually calcium phosphates are in abundance, which means that around 80% are visible on X-rays. Calculi in the distal submandibular (Wharton's) duct can be removed via an oral incision, but submandibular calculi located more proximally usually necessitate removal of the gland. There is also mounting interest in stone removal via sialoendoscopy, a technique that was pioneered in the early 1990s. Ludwig's angina is an infection of the floor of the mouth that can compromise the airway. It usually occurs secondary to disease of the lower third molar teeth, but can also occur secondary to infected sialadenitis.

121. Answers: FFTFF

Barrett's oesophagus is the term used to describe metaplasia of squamous epithelium to intestinal-type columnar epithelium secondary to chronic gastro-oesophageal reflux. It predominantly affects Caucasian males above the age of 50 years. It is considered to be a pre-malignant condition that increases the risk of oesophageal adenocarcinoma. Interventions aim to reduce the degree of acid reflux. In cases of severe dysplasia other treatments include surgery, radiotherapy and laser therapy.

122. Branchial (pharyngeal) cysts:
- Lie along the antero-medial border of the sternocleidomastoid
- Women are twice as likely to be affected
- Usually present as an otherwise asymptomatic neck mass
- Are frequently bilateral
- Should undergo fine-needle aspiration cytology

123. Parathyroid glands:
- Are located on the anterior surface of the thyroid gland
- Produce parathyroid hormone and calcitonin
- Primary hyperparathyroidism leads to hypercalcaemia
- Chronic renal failure is the most common cause of secondary hyperparathyroidism
- Parathyroidectomy is indicated for symptomatic primary hyperparathyroidism

122. Answers: TFTFT

Branchial cysts usually lie along the junction between the upper third and the lower two-thirds of the antero-medial border of the sternoclei-domastoid. The sexes are equally affected. Presentation is usually as an asymptomatic neck mass, although they may present when infected as an inflamed tender neck swelling. Only around 2–3% of branchial cysts are bilateral. Sometimes what appears to be a branchial cyst is actually a cystic squamous-cell metastasis to a cervical lymph node, so suspected branchial cysts should undergo aspiration cytology.

123. Answers: FFTTT

There are usually two paired parathyroid glands (superior and inferior) located on the posterior surface of the thyroid gland. The glands can be either within the fibrous capsule of the thyroid (intracapsular) or outside it (extracapsular). This is surgically relevant, as an intracapsular parathyroid tumour will expand locally within the thyroid capsule, whereas an extracapsular parathyroid tumour may expand downward into the mediastinum. Calcitonin is produced by C-cells of the thyroid gland. Parathyroid hormone has actions on the bone, kidney and intestine which act to increase serum calcium levels. It enhances osteoclast activity, increases active absorption of calcium (and increases phosphate excretion) from the kidney, and enhances absorption of calcium in the intestine by increasing the production of activated vitamin D.

Miscellaneous

124. The following are second pharyngeal arch derivatives:
- The orbicularis oculi muscle
- The arytenoid cartilages
- The stapedius muscle
- The tensor tympani muscle
- The inferior parathyroid glands

125. The following statements about lasers are true:
- Lasers are a form of electromagnetic radiation
- The CO_2 laser is in the visible spectrum of light
- The KTP laser is well absorbed by haemoglobin
- The CO_2 laser is used in laryngeal surgery because of its photo-disruptive effects
- In airway laser surgery, the concentration of oxygen should be maintained above 50%

126. Malignant melanoma:
- Is a malignancy of the Langerhans cells of the skin
- Can be caused by exposure to UVA radiation
- Prognosis is related to tumour depth
- May be cured by surgery alone
- Can occur in the maxillary sinus

124. Answers: TFTFF

The nerve of the second pharyngeal arch is the facial nerve, and so all muscles supplied by that nerve are of second arch origin, including the orbicularis oculi and stapedius muscles, but not the tensor tympani, which is supplied by the mandibular nerve (first arch). The laryngeal cartilages, including the arytenoid, are derived from the fourth and sixth pharyngeal arches. The inferior parathyroid glands are derived from the third pharyngeal arch.

125. Answers: TFTFF

LASER is an acronym for Light Amplification by Stimulated Emission of Radiation, and lasers are a form of electromagnetic radiation. They deliver a focused high-energy source, and have a variety of effects on human tissue, depending upon the energy level used and the duration of exposure. These can be divided into photochemical, photothermal, photodisruptive (plasma ball) and photoablative effects. Photothermal effects predominate in ENT use, including use in the larynx, and photodisruptive effects from high energy should be minimised in order to limit collateral tissue damage. The wavelength of the KTP laser is close to the peak absorption of haemoglobin, so this laser is particularly useful for treating vascular lesions such as those found in hereditary haemorrhagic telangiectasia. The CO_2 laser is invisible and so must be used with a visible aiming beam; it is mainly utilised in laryngeal surgery. In laser airway surgery, oxygen concentrations need to be minimised in order to reduce the risk of airway fire, and levels below 50% should be used.

126. Answers: FTTTT

Melanoma is a malignancy of melanocytes that predominantly occurs in the skin, but can also occur in the eyes, nose, sinuses, meninges, ears, genitals and gastrointestinal tract. Cutaneous melanoma is associated with both UVA and UVB radiation exposure, particularly from strong sunlight or sunbeds. Prognosis is related to depth of tumour invasion, measured histologically by Breslow's depth or Clark's levels. Surgery is the main treatment. Metastatic spread is often treated with chemotherapy or radiotherapy for symptom relief, but these treatments rarely alter survival rates.

127. Fine-needle aspiration cytology (FNAC):
- May be used to diagnose follicular carcinoma of the thyroid
- Fluid from a thyroglossal cyst is rich in cholesterol crystals
- Should only be performed under local anaesthesia
- A Thy 1 result suggests a benign lesion
- Can identify squamous-cell carcinoma

128. Cigarette smoking is associated with an increased risk of:
- Otosclerosis
- Supraglottic carcinoma
- Tonsillar carcinoma
- Thyroid carcinoma
- Reinke's oedema

129. Obstructive sleep apnoea (OSA):
- Is more common in males
- Is associated with Treacher–Collins syndrome
- The gold standard for diagnosis is the Epworth Sleepiness Scale
- May be treated with continuous positive airway pressure (CPAP)
- Is associated with higher mortality

127. Answers: FTFFT
Fine-needle aspiration cytology cannot distinguish follicular adenoma from carcinoma. Classically the fluid aspirated from a thyroglossal cyst is rich in cholesterol crystals. Local anaesthesia is not required for a fine-needle aspiration, but should be used when taking core biopsies. A Thy 1 result means that the sample is inadequate for examination. Where necessary, FNAC can be used to identify the presence of squamous-cell carcinoma in lymph nodes, and so may avoid the need for a lymph node excision biopsy. The latter is best avoided because it could compromise subsequent oncological clearance from a neck dissection.

128. Answers: FTTFT
Cigarette smoking is strongly associated with an increased risk of oral, pharyngeal and laryngeal cancer due to the direct exposure to carcinogens. There is no increased risk of thyroid carcinoma in smokers, and there may actually be a reduced risk. Reinke's oedema is an oedema of the vocal folds, most commonly caused by irritation from cigarette smoke. There is no known association between smoking and otosclerosis.

129. Answers: TTFTT
OSA describes frequent collapse of the upper airway, usually at multiple levels, leading to episodes of reduced airflow (hypopnoea) or total cessation of airflow (apnoea). It is more common in males. Obesity is a major risk factor, but disorders that can decrease the luminal diameter of the upper airway are also associated, including Down syndrome and Treacher–Collins syndrome. The gold standard for diagnosis of OSA is polysomnography, but the Epworth Sleepiness Scale is a sensitive screening test to find those who warrant further investigation. OSA is associated with an increased risk of all-cause mortality, diabetes and cardiovascular disease. The risk is reduced with treatment, and the mainstay of treatment is continuous positive airway pressure (CPAP), with surgery to refashion the upper airway reserved for a few select cases.

130. Basal-cell carcinoma:
- Is the most common skin malignancy
- Arises from cells of the dermis
- Occurs more frequently in individuals with red hair
- Metastasises early
- Is sensitive to chemotherapy

131. The following are risk factors for oesophageal squamous-cell carcinoma:
- Smoking
- Gastro-oesophageal reflux disease
- Plummer–Vinson (Paterson–Brown-Kelly) syndrome
- Multiple endocrine neoplasia (MEN) type 2B
- Multiple endocrine neoplasia (MEN) type 1

132. ENT complications of haematoma include:
- Relapsing polychondritis
- Infection
- Saddle-nose deformity
- Bat ear
- Airway obstruction

130. Answers: TFTFF

Basal-cell carcinoma (BCC) accounts for around 85% of skin malignancy, but very few deaths: it is locally invasive but rarely metastasises. It arises from the basal cells of the epidermis. The main risk factor is exposure to ultraviolet (UV) radiation, especially UVB radiation from sunlight. Fitzpatrick skin type 1 (very white or freckled skin that easily burns and never tans) commonly occurs in individuals with red hair, and this is the skin type with the highest risk of developing BCC. Treatment involves surgical excision, but radiotherapy may be used as an adjunct or for palliative treatment. Chemotherapy has no role.

131. Answers: TFTFF

The main risk factors for squamous-cell carcinoma of the oesophagus are smoking and alcohol consumption. The rare Plummer–Vinson syndrome (a triad of post-cricoid oesophageal webs, glossitis and iron-deficiency anaemia) is also a risk factor. Gastro-oesophageal reflux is a risk factor in the development of adenocarcinoma of the oesophagus, usually in the lower oesophagus, against a background of metaplasia (Barrett's oesophagus). Multiple endocrine neoplasia has no association with oesophageal carcinoma, as the oesophagus has no endocrine tissue.

132. Answers: FTTFT

Haematoma usually occurs following trauma, including surgery. Haematoma on the nasal septum can lead to septal cartilage necrosis and consequent saddle-nose deformity. Cartilage necrosis from haematoma of the pinna can cause a cauliflower ear deformity, but not bat ear, which is a congenital deformity. A large haematoma in the neck (e.g. from trauma or following thyroid surgery) can compress the trachea to cause airway compromise. Any haematoma can become infected. Relapsing polychondritis is an autoimmune disorder of uncertain cause, but not a complication of haematoma formation.

133. Evidence-based medicine (EBM):
- Involves formulating a clearly defined question
- Treatments should only be recommended if there is a randomised trial to confirm their efficacy
- Began in the 1980s
- Level Ia evidence refers to a randomised placebo-controlled trial
- Will always confirm or refute the efficacy of a treatment

134. Local anaesthetics:
- Act by increasing the membrane permaeability of nerve fibres to sodium
- Lignocaine is shorter acting than bupivacaine
- Lignocaine works better under acidic conditions
- Adrenaline may help to increase the duration of anaesthesia
- 1% lignocaine solution contains 1 mg/ml of lignocaine

135. Wound healing may be impaired by:
- Infection
- Previous radiotherapy
- Raised vitamin C levels
- Low zinc levels
- Age

133. Answers: TFFFF

Evidence-based medicine is the conscientious, explicit and judicious use of current best evidence when making decisions about the individual care of patients. It has been practised for centuries, and some have traced its origins to ancient Greece or ancient China, although the term 'evidence-based medicine' was only coined in 1990. There should be a clearly defined question to be answered. It is important to remember that the aim is to apply the best available evidence to clinical practice, but this may not necessarily be high-level evidence. When the principles of evidence-based medicine are applied, it is not unusual to be in a position where you conclude that there is insufficient evidence to either support or refute a treatment. Level Ia evidence refers to a systematic review or meta-analysis of randomised controlled trials.

134. Answers: FTFTF

Local anaesthetic agents act by reducing the membrane permeability of nerve fibres to sodium. Lignocaine is an example of a short-acting local anaesthetic, and bupivacaine is an example of a long-acting one. Local anaesthetics are weak bases and so work better at a higher pH, at which they are less ionised. The addition of adrenaline to an anaesthetic infiltration helps to prolong the duration of effect because vasoconstriction reduces clearance. This also allows the use of a higher total dose of local anaesthetic (e.g. from 3 mg/kg of lignocaine to 7 mg/kg of lignocaine with adrenaline). 1% lignocaine solution contains 10 mg/ml of lignocaine.

135. Answers: TTFTT

Many factors can affect wound healing. Infection lowers local oxygen tension, is collagenolytic, and inhibits re-epithelialisation. Radiotherapy can cause an obliterative endarteritis with chronic tissue hypoxia around a wound. The elderly heal less well than the young, with regard to both the speed of healing and the tensile strength of the wound. Low levels of zinc, copper or magnesium can be detrimental to healing, because they are cofactors for enzymes in repair mechanisms. A deficiency of vitamin A or vitamin C can also impair healing because these compounds are required for collagen synthesis and modification. Drugs such as steroids, NSAIDs and anti-neoplastic agents may also delay healing.

136. The following statistical tests are intended for data that show a Gaussian (normal) distribution:
- Mann–Whitney test
- One-sample *t*-test
- Chi-squared test
- Mean
- Wilcoxon test

137. Surgical sutures:
- A braided suture has a higher risk of wound infection than a monofilament suture
- Sutures should be tied as tightly as possible
- An interrupted suture should be avoided following thyroidectomy
- A 6/0 suture is suitable for closing a parotidectomy incision
- Absorbable sutures are contraindicated for skin closure

138. Consent:
- Informed consent requires the patient to believe the information that is presented to them
- Consent for a surgical procedure is only valid for a period of 3 months
- Only complications that occur in more than 1% of cases are relevant
- Consent forms should be counter-signed by the responsible consultant
- A parent/guardian is required to sign the consent form for patients under 18 years of age

136. Answers: FTFTF

The Gaussian or normal distribution describes a bell-shaped distribution of values that is valid for many continuous biological traits (e.g. height, intelligence, serum albumin concentration). When data are more or less normally distributed, parametric statistical tests can be used. Non-parametric tests must be used for data that are not normally distributed. Parametric tests include the mean (the total of all values divided by the number of values, which usually corresponds to the peak of the bell curve) and the t-test (for comparing groups, which includes the paired t-test for comparing paired groups, the unpaired t-test for comparing unpaired groups, and the one-sample t-test for comparing with a hypothetical value). Data that are not normally distributed can be ranked; the median is then a good measure of the average, and the Mann–Whitney test is used to compare unpaired groups and the Wilcoxon test is used to compare paired groups. The Chi-squared test is used to compare groups with a binomial outcome (e.g. Yes/No), and so is also a non-parametric test. Many other parametric and non-parametric statistical tests are available for use in specified circumstances.

137. Answers: TFFFF

Sutures can be classified as monofilament or polyfilament/braided, and as absorbable or non-absorbable. Suture diameter is classified according to the *United States Pharmacopeia* classification, which originally classified sutures on a scale of 1 to 6, with 1 being the thinnest. With improvements in manufacturing, increasingly thin sutures became possible, allowing the production of '0' suture, '00' (2–0) suture, '000' (3–0) suture, etc. 6/0 suture is too weak for a parotidectomy wound, for which 3–0 would be more suitable. Braided sutures are at higher risk of infection than monofilament sutures because bacteria can become trapped between the braids. Sutures should be tied tight enough to hold the wound edges in close apposition, but not too tight, as this may cause tissue ischaemia. Sutures may be tied interrupted or continuously. Interrupted sutures are considered to be preferable to continuous sutures following thyroidectomy because if there is post-operative haemorrhage the wound may need to be quickly opened to prevent compression of the airway by haematoma. Non-absorbable sutures are used for skin closure because they are less antigenic. They do need to be removed (e.g. 5–7 days later), but this means that all foreign material is removed from the wound at this stage. However, there is no absolute contraindication to the use of absorbable sutures for skin closure, especially modern monofilament absorbable sutures.

138. Answers: TFFFF

The conditions for informed consent are that information that is delivered to the patient should be believed, understood and retained. There is no time limit for the validity of consent. However, a common-sense approach is advisable, and if there is a significant time lapse between consent and surgery, the surgeon has a responsibility to discuss options closer to the time. The idea that only risks which occur in more than 1% of cases need to be discussed is erroneous. Potential complications that may incur severe morbidity or even mortality must be explained even if they occur in less than 1% of cases. A good rule of thumb is to explain to the patient what you would want to know if you were about to undergo this procedure yourself. A parent or guardian is required to provide consent for children under the age of 16 years, although 'Gillick' competency may be assumed for those under 16 years in exceptional circumstances.

139. The following are autoimmune diseases:
- Seasonal allergic rhinitis
- Relapsing polychondritis
- Thyroid eye disease
- Glandular fever
- Eagle syndrome

140. Orbital blow-out fractures:
- Are usually caused by blunt non-penetrating trauma to the globe
- There is classically an upward and medial displacement of the eye
- Signs include enophthalmos and diplopia
- Forced duction testing is a useful assessment
- Extra-ocular muscle entrapment is an indication for surgical repair

141. In laryngopharyngeal carcinoma, histological features that predict a worse outcome include:
- Cervical metastases
- Extra-capsular spread of tumour
- Spindle-cell variant
- Presence of human papilloma virus
- Perineural invasion

139. Answers: FTTFF

Seasonal allergic rhinitis is a type 1 hypersensitivity reaction to an exogenous antigen, namely pollen. Relapsing polychondritis is thought to be an autoimmune disease, with antibodies to cartilage types II, IX and XI found in 50% of patients. Thyroid eye disease is thought to occur due to autoantibodies to the TSH receptor which cross-react with intra-orbital elements. Glandular fever is caused by Epstein–Barr virus and is not autoimmune. Eagle syndrome is a rare anatomical anomaly in which a prolonged styloid process impinges on local structures, typically causing pain.

140. Answers: TFTTT

Orbital blow-out fracture is caused by a blunt, non-penetrating missile that strikes the globe and causes a sudden increase in intra-orbital pressure. The orbital floor fractures into the maxillary sinus, or the medial orbital wall may fracture into the ethmoid sinuses. Enophthalmos and diplopia may be observed due to downward displacement of the globe and entrapment of the extra-ocular muscles (particularly the inferior rectus). Forced duction testing can be performed under local or general anaesthetic, and involves examining for extra-ocular muscle entrapment. Enophthalmos and extra-ocular muscle entrapment are indications for surgical repair.

141. Answers: TTTFT

Cervical metastasis is the most important prognostic factor in head and neck cancer, as it signifies not only that the disease has metastatic potential, but also that this potential has been realised. Extra-capsular spread on histology is a further sign of metastatic potential, and further reduces the prognosis by 50%. Spindle-cell or basaloid-cell tumours behave more aggressively than papillary or verrucous forms. Perineural invasion predicts local recurrence and carries a worse prognosis. Oropharyngeal carcinomas associated with HPV infection carry a better prognosis than those associated with tobacco and alcohol exposure.

142. The following agents are commonly used to treat head and neck carcinoma:
- Cetuximab
- Melphalan
- Vincristine
- Cisplatin
- Azathioprine

143. Signs found in hypovolaemic shock include:
- Tachypnoea
- Capillary refill time of more than 3 seconds
- Increased urine output
- Normal blood pressure
- Low blood pressure

144. In the normal infant:
- The circulating blood volume is approximately 50 ml/kg
- The glottis is the narrowest part of the airway
- Aspirin is a good choice of analgesic
- Parental consent is not always required for treatment
- A respiratory rate of 40 breaths per minute is within the normal range

142. Answers: TFFTF

Chemotherapy has been shown to improve survival in locally advanced head and neck cancer when used with other measures such as surgery or radiotherapy. Platinum-based compounds which cross-link DNA, such as cisplatin, are most commonly used. Cetuximab is an epidermal growth factor receptor inhibitor which has also been shown to improve survival. It is used in patients who are unable to tolerate conventional chemotherapy. Melphalan is used to treat multiple myeloma and ovarian cancer. Vincristine is used in lymphoma, acute lymphoblastic leukaemia and nephroblastoma. Azathioprine is an immunosuppressant agent. It may increase the risk of certain cancers, but has no role in their treatment.

143. Answers: TTFTT

Shock is a state of reduced tissue and organ perfusion. Where this is due to decreased circulating blood volume, it is known as hypovolaemic shock. Hypovolaemic shock has four stages. In stage 1 (< 15% volume loss) there may be few signs other than pallor, and vasoconstriction maintains blood pressure. In stage 2 (15–30% volume loss), vasconstriction alone can no longer maintain cardiac output, and there is a reduced diastolic blood pressure, tachycardia, tachypnoea and sweating. In stage 3 (30–40% volume loss), systolic blood pressure also falls and there is marked tachypnoea and tachycardia, with an agitated mental state, pallor and sweating. In stage 4 (> 40% volume loss), systolic pressure falls further, giving a weak pulse, extreme tachycardia and tachypnoea and reduced conscious level. As blood volume decreases, perfusion shifts from the periphery to the central organs, leading to a capillary refill time that is longer than the normal value of less than 2 seconds. In addition, the renin–angiotensin system is activated by reduced perfusion of the kidneys, leading to reabsorption of sodium and water to conserve intravascular volume, thereby reducing urine output.

144. Answers: FFFTT

The normal blood volume of a child is 75–80 ml/kg. The cricoid cartilage is the narrowest part of the airway. Aspirin should be avoided in children because of the risk of Reye syndrome, namely inflammation of organs (especially the brain and liver) of uncertain aetiology. Treatment should be with parental consent where possible, but in an emergency situation parental consent is not legally required if one is acting in the best interests of the child. The normal respiratory rate of an infant is 30–60 breaths per minute, and the normal pulse rate is 100–160 beats per minute.

145. Oral steroids are a beneficial treatment for:
- Bell's palsy
- Subglottic haemangioma
- Post-tonsillectomy analgesia
- Pharyngeal pouch
- Allergic rhinitis

146. Facial plastics:
- Incisions should run perpendicular to relaxed skin tension lines
- Monofilament sutures are preferable for skin closure
- Z-plasty may be used to improve the appearance of scars
- Keloid scars should be treated with surgical excision in the first instance
- Hypertrophic scarring has a later onset compared with keloid scars

147. Wegener's granulomatosis:
- Most commonly involves the nose
- More commonly affects the Caucasian population
- Is a common cause of bony septal perforation
- May be diagnosed by nasal biopsy
- Corticosteroids are a recognised treatment

145. Answers: TTTFT

Steroids are theoretically useful in the treatment of any inflammatory disorder, but significant benefit has been clearly demonstrated only in certain diseases. Recent large-scale studies have shown that steroids improve long-term recovery from Bell's palsy. They can also significantly reduce the size of subglottic haemangioma, although reported success rates vary between 10% and 90%. The mechanism of haemangioma formation is uncertain, but does involve inflammatory mediators. Several studies show better analgesia following tonsillectomy with steroids. Severe allergic rhinitis can be treated with short courses of systemic steroids if, for example, symptomatic relief is required for an important life event. Steroids have no role in the treatment of pharyngeal pouch.

146. Answers: FTTFF

Relaxed skin tension lines generally lie perpendicular to the underlying facial musculature. Incisions should be made parallel to the tension lines in order to minimise scarring. Skin closure is best carried out using monofilament sutures, which have less tissue reactivity and a lower incidence of wound infection. Z-plasty is a technique that may be particularly useful for realigning distorted anatomical areas. Keloid scars differ from hypertrophic scars in that they extend beyond the original scar margin. Keloid scars generally have a later onset, and may appear up to 1 year after the original incision. Conservative and medical therapy is generally considered before electing for surgical excision of keloid scarring. Recurrence following surgical excision may occur, and may be worse than the original lesion.

147. Answers: FFFTT

Wegener's granulomatosis is a systemic vasculitis that primarily involves the lungs and kidneys, but also commonly affects the upper respiratory tract. There is no predilection for the Caucasian race. Granulomatous disease in the nose usually causes cartilaginous destruction rather than bony septal perforation. Nasal biopsy may provide the diagnosis, although renal biopsy usually has a greater diagnostic yield. Immunosuppressant therapies such as corticosteroids, cyclophosphamide and azathioprine may be used to treat Wegener's granulomatosis, depending upon the severity of the disease. The antibiotic co-trimoxazole has recently been shown to be of benefit in reducing relapse rates.

148. Down syndrome is associated with:
- Otitis media with effusion
- Congenital sensorineural hearing loss
- Obstructive sleep apnoea
- Hypothyroidism
- Tracheomalacia

149. Clinical trials:
- Absolute risk reduction is the risk in the treated group minus the risk in the control group
- A P-value below 0.05 means that the probability of a result occurring by chance is less than 1 in 20
- A study has a type II error if there is a failure to reject the null hypothesis when the null hypothesis is false
- An intention-to-treat analysis helps to limit crossover and drop-out bias
- A randomised placebo-controlled trial will provide type Ia evidence

150. Imaging:
- CT is more useful than MRI for delineating bony anatomy
- Ultrasound may distinguish between cystic and solid lesions
- A lateral X-ray of the neck is a useful early investigation in the diagnosis of epiglottitis
- Barium swallow is useful for identifying the cause of aspiration
- CT is contraindicated in patients with cardiac pacemakers

148. Answers: TTTTT

Down syndrome has numerous ENT manifestations. Children with Down syndrome may suffer from conductive hearing loss due to otitis media with effusion, or from congenital sensorineural loss. Therefore all children with Down syndrome should have an objective test of hearing early in life. There is an increased risk of obstructive sleep apnoea due to reduced nasopharyngeal dimensions from midface hypoplasia, combined with general hypotonicity. There is also a higher incidence of tracheomalacia and cardiac defects. Hypothyroidism is more common in Down syndrome, and may be difficult to identify clinically because hypothyroid facies may be masked by the other facial dysmorphology.

149. Answers: FTTTF

Absolute risk reduction refers to the risk in the control group minus the risk in the treated group. It may also be described as the inverse of the number needed to treat (i.e. ARR = 1/NNT). A type I error refers to a false positive, and involves rejecting the null hypothesis when the null hypothesis is true. A type II error refers to a false negative, and involves failing to reject the null hypothesis when the null hypothesis is false. An intention-to-treat analysis involves analysing patient outcomes according to the original groups to which the patients were assigned, rather than the actual treatment received. This helps to limit crossover and dropout bias. Level Ia evidence refers to a systematic review of randomised controlled trials.

150. Answers: TTFFF

In general CT is more useful for delineating bony anatomy, whereas MRI shows better visualisation of soft tissues. Ultrasound may distinguish between cystic and solid lesions, and has the benefit of no exposure to radiation. Acute epiglottitis is a medical emergency, and a clinical diagnosis and management should not be delayed by radiology. The 'thumbprint' sign of epiglottitis may be seen on a lateral cervical spine X-ray, and results from a thickened free edge of the epiglottis. Video-fluoroscopy with water-soluble contrast media can be useful in the investigation of aspiration, but barium must be avoided, as aspiration into the lung will result in a chemical pneumonitis. MRI is relatively contraindicated in patients with a cardiac pacemaker, but local protocols should be consulted, as sometimes MRI can be performed under carefully controlled conditions. There is no contraindication to the use of CT with cardiac pacemakers.

Extended Matching Questions (EMQs)

Otology

1. Sensorineural hearing loss:

   A Ménière disease

   B Noise-induced hearing loss

   C Presbycusis

   D Genetic (familial) hearing loss

   E Vestibular schwannoma (acoustic neuroma)

   F Meningitis

   G Ototoxicity

   For each of the following clinical scenarios, select the probable cause of hearing loss:

   1 A 30-year-old woman presents with gradual-onset hearing loss. The audiogram shows bilateral sensorineural hearing loss with thresholds of 40 dB across all frequencies. There is no history of vertigo.

   2 A 53-year-old man presents with sudden hearing loss in the left ear. He is otherwise asymptomatic. The audiogram shows a left dead ear.

   3 An 83-year-old man presents with gradual-onset hearing loss. The audiogram shows down-sloping bilateral sensorineural hearing loss.

2. Conductive hearing loss:

   A Otosclerosis

   B Acute suppurative otitis media

   C Otitis media with effusion (glue ear)

   D Tympanosclerosis

   E Ossicular erosion

   F Ossicular dislocation

   G Perilymph fistula

   For each of the following clinical scenarios, select the probable cause of hearing loss:

   1 A 35-year-old woman presents with a gradual onset of hearing loss in her left ear. The audiogram shows a left conductive hearing loss with an air–bone gap of 20 dB across all frequencies, but with air–bone closure at 4 kHz. The tympanogram shows a type A trace.

   2 A 52-year-old man presents with a hearing loss in the left ear following an upper respiratory tract infection. He has no otalgia.

   3 A 36-year-old man is involved in a road traffic accident with significant head injury. When he regains consciousness he has a unilateral hearing loss. The audiogram shows a 60 dB conductive hearing loss across all frequencies.

1. Answers: 1D 2E 3C

Mid-frequency hearing loss is typically due to genetic changes (most of which have not been classified), but it is important to remember that other causes of hearing loss also have a significant genetic predisposition (e.g. noise-induced hearing loss or presbycusis). In most cases of sudden hearing loss the cause is uncertain and may be related to cochlear ischaemia or viral infection, but a vestibular schwannoma should be excluded by MRI imaging. Presbycusis is a term used to describe age-related hearing loss that is probably multi-factorial, but which typically causes a down-sloping high-frequency sensorineural hearing loss.

2. Answers: 1A 2C 3F

Otosclerosis causes a conductive hearing loss, typically with a Carhart notch at 4 kHz. The tympanogram is normal. Both acute suppurative otitis media and a middle ear effusion may follow an upper respiratory tract infection, but the absence of otalgia in this case makes the latter more likely. Significant head injury can cause a sensorineural hearing loss through cochlear concussion or fracture, but may also cause a conductive hearing loss by dislocation of the ossicles. A maximal conductive hearing loss will consequently occur, which is 60 dB across all frequencies.

3. Dizziness:

   A Benign paroxysmal positional vertigo

   B Central dysfunction

   C Ménière disease

   D Vestibular neuronitis/labyrinthitis

   E Labyrinthine fistula

   F Vestibular schwannoma (acoustic neuroma)

   G Vertebro-basilar ischaemia

   H Psychiatric disease

   For each of the following clinical scenarios, select the most likely cause of dizziness:

   1 A 42-year-old woman who over the last 4 years has had three attacks of debilitating vertigo lasting a few hours, each time preceded by aural fullness and tinnitus in the left ear.

   2 A 68-year-old man who has become progressively unsteady with occasional vertigo. He has tinnitus in the right ear, and the audiogram shows an asymmetrical high-frequency sensorineural hearing loss in the right ear.

   3 An 82-year-old woman who has a 2-month history of vertiginous spells when turning over in bed. These episodes last only a few seconds. The audiogram shows a symmetrical bilateral high-frequency sensorineural hearing loss.

   4 A 32-year-old man who has become progressively ataxic. He displays nystagmus on lateral and upward gaze. The audiogram is normal.

4. Audiological investigations:

   A Pure-tone audiogram

   B Tympanogram

   C Auditory brainstem response

   D Play audiogram

   E Speech audiogram

   F Oto-acoustic emissions

   G Stenger test

   H Caloric testing

   Select the most appropriate audiological investigation for each of the following scenarios:

   1 A 3-year-old boy whose parents have expressed concerns about his hearing.

   2 A newborn child who has two deaf parents.

   3 A 7-month-old, apparently deaf girl who is being considered for a cochlear implant.

   4 A 7-year-old boy who says that he can't hear the teacher.

3. Answers: 1C 2F 3A 4B

The diagnosis of dizziness is largely based upon the history; investigation is rarely helpful. Repeated attacks of debilitating vertigo with synchronous hearing loss, tinnitus and aural fullness are suggestive of Ménière disease. Vestibular schwannoma can cause dizziness, and the symptoms of unilateral tinnitus and an asymmetrical hearing loss should make one suspect this as a cause. The history given for BPPV is almost pathognomonic; the audiogram in this patient is what would be expected from presbycusis. Progressive ataxia raises a suspicion of central disease, and vertical nystagmus makes this diagnosis highly likely.

4. Answers: 1D 2F 3C 4A

The pure-tone audiogram is the most useful preliminary test of hearing in adults and older children (typically those above the age of 5 years). Play audiometry may be used for younger children, from around the age of 3 years. Oto-acoustic emissions are now used for universal neonatal screening of hearing in the UK. A young child who is being considered for cochlear implantation requires an accurate assessment of hearing thresholds. This can be difficult in the very young, so auditory brainstem response (under general anaesthetic) is often used to provide an objective assessment.

5. Syndromic hearing loss:
   A Neurofibromatosis type 2   F Waardenburg syndrome
   B Jervell and Lange–Nielsen   G Seckel syndrome
     syndrome
   C Pendred syndrome   H Refsum syndrome
   D Usher syndrome   I Hersh syndrome
   E Alport syndrome

   For each of the following clinical scenarios, identify the likely syndromic cause of sensorineural deafness:
   1 A child born profoundly deaf with an enlarged thyroid
   2 A child with a white forelock born with a moderate hearing loss
   3 A child with haematuria who develops gradual high-frequency hearing loss
   4 A child born profoundly deaf who has cardiac arrhythmia

6. Treatment of hearing loss:
   A No treatment   E Grommet (ventilation tube)
   B Conventional hearing aid   F Cochlear implant
   C Bone-anchored hearing   G Auditory brainstem implant
     aid
   D Ossicular surgery

   For each of the following conditions, select the most appropriate treatment:
   1 During a routine employment screen, a 40-year-old woman is found to have a 10 dB air–bone gap in the right ear with a Carhart notch. The tympanogram is type A. She has no hearing disability.
   2 A 42-year-old man with neurofibromatosis type 2 has had bilateral large vestibular schwannomas (acoustic neuromas) resected.

5.   Answers: 1C 2F 3E 4B

There are many genetic causes of deafness, some of which are syndromic. Pendred syndrome is associated with goitre and sometimes with hyperthyroidism. Waardenburg syndrome is characterised by a variable degree of hearing loss and neural crest and pigmentation defects such as heterochromia iridis, hypertelorism and a white forelock. Alport syndrome is associated with a high-frequency hearing loss and glomerulonephritis and ocular abnormalities. Jervell and Lange–Nielsen syndrome is caused by a defect in a potassium channel leading to deafness and a prolonged cardiac QT interval.

6.   Answers: 1A 2G

The woman in the first scenario probably has previously undiagnosed otosclerosis. As it is unilateral, mild and, most importantly, is not causing disability, no treatment is required. The man who has had bilateral vestibular schwannoma excision will not have any auditory nerves to convey signals to the brainstem. Therefore he can only be aided with an auditory brainstem implant.

7. Otalgia:

A Chronic suppurative otitis media

B Cholesteatoma

C Fungal otitis externa

D Referred pain

E Ramsay Hunt syndrome

F Vestibular schwannoma

G Malignant otitis externa

H Foreign body in ear

For each of the following clinical scenarios, select the most likely diagnosis:

1 A 64-year-old diabetic patient presents with severe otalgia that is unrelieved by oral paracetamol, diclofenac and oral morphine solution. Examination of the ear is exquisitely painful and shows granulation tissue in the external auditory canal, but minimal debris.

2 A 45-year-old patient presents with a severe dull pain within the right ear that has radiated to include the pinna. The patient reports a ringing in the ears. On examination there are small blisters over the auricle and within the external auditory canal. The patient has some difficulty in closing the right eye.

8. Tuning fork tests:

A Left conductive hearing loss

B Right sensorineural hearing loss

C Right conductive hearing loss

D Bilateral conductive hearing loss

E Bilateral sensorineural hearing loss

F Left sensorineural hearing loss

G Right hyperacusis

H Left hyperacusis

Select the most likely diagnosis for each of the following tuning fork examination scenarios:

1 Weber test localises to the right side. Rinne test is positive on the left and right side.

2 Weber test localises to the right side. Rinne test is negative on the right side and positive on the left side.

7. Answers: 1G 2E

Malignant otitis externa results from the spread of infection to cause an osteitis of the temporal bone. Infection can track along the skull base, giving rise to cranial nerve palsies. Patients who are immunocompromised (e.g. diabetics) are at greater risk, and *Pseudomonas* species are often isolated. It is particularly important to consider this diagnosis when a patient presents with otalgia that seems to be excessive compared with the findings on clinical examination. Treatment involves intravenous antibiotic therapy and also surgical debridement in some cases. The patient will require a protracted course of oral antibiotic therapy after the initial aggressive management. Ramsay Hunt syndrome results from herpes zoster reactivation within the geniculate ganglion of the facial nerve. The patient often complains of severe otalgia with a vesicular rash over the external ear and auditory canal (in the distribution of the nervus intermedius). Due to the communications of the facial nerve, the soft palate and tongue may be involved. Involvement of motor branches causes facial weakness. There may also be sensorineural hearing loss and tinnitus. Aciclovir or valciclovir with steroids is the treatment of choice.

8. Answers: 1F 2C

The Weber and Rinne tuning fork tests are a useful means of audiological assessment in the clinic and at the bedside. The Weber test is particularly useful for identifying a unilateral hearing loss. It compares bone conduction in both ears such that if a conductive loss of 10 dB or more is present, the sound is heard in the affected ear (i.e. it lateralises to the affected ear). If there is a sensorineural hearing loss in the contralateral ear, the sound will localise to the normal ear. The Rinne test compares the ability of the patient to hear a tone conducted via air and bone in each ear. If air conduction is better than bone conduction, the ear is normal or there is a sensorineural impairment (i.e. air conduction and bone conduction are reduced equally). This is a Rinne positive result. If bone conduction is greater than air conduction, there is a conductive hearing loss. This is a Rinne negative result.

9. Hearing aids:

    A Bone-anchored hearing   E In-the-canal hearing aid
       aid (BAHA)
    B Cochlear implant   F Auditory brainstem implant
    C Ventilation tube   G CROS hearing aid
    D Behind-the-ear hearing aid

    For each of the following scenarios, select the most appropriate
    method of hearing treatment:
    1 A 62-year-old patient suffering from bilateral chronic otitis
       externa with a bilateral mixed hearing loss.
    2 A 34-year-old woman with bilateral mild to moderate sen-
       sorineural hearing loss who feels embarrassed about using a
       readily visible hearing aid at work.

10. Congenital hearing loss:

    A Crouzon syndrome   F Waardenburg syndrome
    B Jervell and Lange–Nielsen   G Pierre Robin sequence
       syndrome
    C Pendred syndrome   H Refsum syndrome
    D Usher syndrome   I Treacher–Collins syndrome
    E Apert syndrome

    For each of the following scenarios, select the most likely diagnosis:
    1 A 2-year-old child with a hypoplastic mandible, cleft palate and
       posterior displacement of the tongue presents with conductive
       hearing loss.
    2 A patient with retinitis pigmentosa and sensorineural hearing
       loss.

9.   Answers: 1A 2E

A bone-anchored hearing aid (BAHA) is a semi-implantable hearing device that relies on direct transmission of mechanical vibrations through the bone of the skull to the cochlea. In the above scenario there is a hearing loss where conventional hearing aids are likely to be problematic due to the persistent infection. Patients with external ear deformities (e.g. microtia) may also benefit from a BAHA. Patients with a unilateral severe hearing loss that has not been helped by traditional hearing aids may also benefit from BAHAs. In-the-canal (ITC) or completely-in-canal (CIC) hearing aids are useful for patients who are particularly self-conscious about wearing a hearing aid. They are not suitable for patients with a severe hearing impairment, as they have limited power.

10.   Answers: 1G 2D

Pierre Robin sequence is the association of micrognathia, cleft palate and glossoptosis (posterior displacement of the tongue). The presence of a cleft palate makes middle ear effusions likely. Usher syndrome is an autosomal-recessive inherited condition which occurs in around 15% of patients with retinitis pigmentosa. The hearing loss is due to degeneration of sensory epithelium and hair cell dysfunction.

11. Tinnitus:

A Noise-induced hearing loss
B Cholesteatoma
C Psychosomatic
D Presbycusis
E Ramsay Hunt syndrome
F Vestibular schwannoma
G Glomus tumour
H Chronic suppurative otitis media

For each of the following clinical scenarios, select the most likely diagnosis:

1 A 65-year-old patient presents with a mild buzzing sound in both ears which is most noticeable at night. He also reports long-standing hearing impairment. A pure-tone audiogram shows bilateral sensorineural hearing loss that is worse in the higher frequencies.

2 A 55-year-old woman presents with a unilateral conductive hearing loss and pulsatile tinnitus in the right ear. Otoscopy reveals a reddish-blue appearance to the tympanic membrane.

12. Management of ear disease:

A Topical olive oil
B Combined-approach tympanoplasty
C Topical aminoglycoside drops
D Topical steroid drops
E Intravenous antibiotics with or without cortical mastoidectomy
F Watch and wait
G Oral amoxicillin
H EUA postnasal space and insertion ventilation tube

For each of the following scenarios, select the appropriate management:

1 A 4-year-old boy is brought to the emergency department with otalgia and discharge from the right ear. His temperature is 39°C. On examination, the right ear appears to be pushed forward.

2 A 40-year-old man presents with a history of unilateral offensive ear discharge for 6 months with squamous debris in the attic (epitympanum) that is not self-cleaning.

11.   Answers: 1D 2G

Presbycusis (age-related hearing loss) may be associated with tinnitus at the frequencies that are worst affected by the hearing impairment. In some cases, conventional hearing aids may improve the tinnitus. The mechanism is unclear, but it has been suggested that amplification of external sounds and improved auditory input may enhance central mechanisms of habituation and promote central adaptive plasticity. Glomus tumours of the temporal bone are rare slow-growing vascular tumours that occur in the region of the jugular bulb and middle ear. The condition usually presents late, but early signs include a conductive hearing loss and a tinnitus that is pulsatile in nature. Involvement of the jugular foramen may result in cranial nerve palsies (IX–XI). Otoscopic examination may reveal the vascular tumour as a reddish-blue mass behind the tympanic membrane.

12.   Answers: 1E 2B

Acute mastoiditis is a medical emergency. It is a complication of acute otitis media that is less common now with the widespread availability of antibiotic therapy. The condition presents as persistent acute otitis media. There may be a post-auricular fluctuant mass with overlying oedema and erythema due to subperiosteal abscess. This displaces the ear outward and forward. Principles of management include intravenous antibiotics with or without cortical mastoidectomy to drain infection. The squamous debris in the attic described in the second scenario is cholesteatoma, which is treated surgically. There are a number of approaches. Canal-wall-up and canal-wall-down procedures (preserving or removing the posterior external auditory canal wall, respectively) may be used according to the preferences of the patient and the surgeon. Combined-approach tympanoplasty is one of the most popular canal-wall-up procedures. The disadvantage of this technique is that the middle ear must be re-opened a few months later to identify any residual disease.

Rhinology and laryngology

13. Control of epistaxis:

A Ascending pharyngeal artery ligation

B Silver nitrate cautery to Little's area

C Greater palatine artery ligation

D Maxillary artery ligation

E External carotid artery ligation

F Sphenopalatine artery ligation

G Posterior ethmoidal artery ligation

H Superior labial artery ligation

I Anterior ethmoidal artery ligation

Select the most appropriate treatment strategy for each of the following clinical scenarios:

1 A 63-year-old patient presents with recurrent epistaxis. On examination, bleeding points are visible on the right anterior nasal septum around 1 cm from the columella.

2 A 24-year-old man presents with severe epistaxis following a punch to the nasal bridge. Bleeding is occurring from the upper nasal cavity and cannot be controlled with packing.

3 A 56-year-old man with recurrent epistaxis is bleeding heavily through a well-packed nose (ribbon gauze packing bilaterally anteriorly, with posterior Foley catheters).

14. Nasal obstruction:

A Nasal fracture

B Antrochoanal polyp

C Foreign body

D Atrophic rhinitis

E Deviated nasal septum

F Perennial rhinitis

G Nasal polyps

H Allergic rhinitis

I Rhinitis medicamentosa

J Septal haematoma

For each of the following clinical scenarios, select the most likely diagnosis:

1 A 36-year-old patient complains of persistent bilateral nasal obstruction despite regular use of nasal decongestants over a period of several months. On examination he has an excellent bilateral nasal airway.

2 A 42-year-old woman complains of a long history of poor sense of smell and bilateral nasal obstruction. On examination, pale swellings are observed in both nasal cavities.

3 A 28-year-old man presents with unilateral nasal obstruction (on the right side) that is worse on expiration. He also reports some right-sided deafness. Otoscopy shows right middle ear effusion.

13. Answers: 1B 2I 3F

Little's area is a confluence of blood vessels at the anterior–inferior part of the nasal septum that is also known as Kiesselbach's plexus. It consists of anastamoses from the anterior ethmoidal, greater palatine, sphenopalatine and superior labial artery, and lateral nasal branches of the facial artery. This area is a common site for epistaxis, and is amenable to silver nitrate cautery to stop bleeding. The next stage of management is nasal packing, and if that fails, endoscopic sphenopalatine artery ligation should be considered. Anterior ethmoidal artery avulsion should be suspected in the presence of severe uncontrollable epistaxis following anterior facial trauma. Anterior ethmoidal artery ligation may require an external, endoscopic or combined approach.

14. Answers: 1I 2G 3B

Rhinitis medicamentosa (RM) refers to nasal congestion that follows overuse of topical nasal vasoconstrictor decongestants. The pathophysiology of RM is unknown, although down-regulation of the involved sympathetic receptors resulting in rebound nasal congestion is a popular theory. Treatment involves abstinence from decongestants, although this may be difficult in some patients, as a degree of psychological dependence may develop. Nasal polyposis can be diagnosed in most cases on clinical examination with anterior rhinoscopy alone. Inflammatory polyps of chronic rhinosinusitis are bilateral and associated with nasal obstruction and hyposmia. Unilateral polypoid disease is a red flag and merits biopsy to exclude malignancy. An antrochoanal polyp is a benign solitary polypoid lesion which usually arises from the maxillary sinus and then enlarges, passing through the sinus ostium into the choana and nasopharynx. Classically there may be a valve effect with nasal obstruction that is worse on expiration. In this case there may be obstruction of the Eustachian tube giving rise to the middle ear effusion. Treatment is by surgical excision.

15. Rhinorrhoea:

A Foreign body
B Seasonal allergic rhinitis
C Common cold
D Cerebrospinal fluid leak
E Chronic rhinosinusitis
F Perennial allergic rhinitis
G Atrophic rhinitis
H Juvenile angiosarcoma
I Nasopharyngeal carcinoma

For each of the following clinical scenarios, select the most likely cause of nasal discharge:

1 A 45-year-old patient presents to the ENT clinic with a history of several months of persistent clear unilateral nasal discharge which began a few weeks after sinus surgery.

2 An anxious parent brings a 5-year-old child to the emergency department with a 2-day history of foul-smelling unilateral nasal discharge.

3 A 14-year-old student complains of itchy eyes, rhinorrhoea and persistent sneezing during the summer term at school.

16. Staging of laryngeal carcinoma:

A T3 N3 Mx
B T1b N2 Mx
C T2 N1 Mx
D T2b N2 Mx
E T3 N2 Mx
F T4 N2b Mx
G T4 N3 M0

Stage each of the following tumours:

1 An examination under anaesthesia of a 55-year-old smoker reveals a squamous-cell carcinoma of the right vocal cord. There is limited movement of the right vocal cord, and a 2 cm lymph node in the right level II neck.

2 A 62-year-old woman presents with a well-differentiated tumour arising from the anterior commissure. CT imaging shows erosion of the thyroid cartilage. There are three 2.5 cm lymph nodes in the left level II neck.

15. Answers: 1D 2A 3B

Unilateral rhinorrhoea following sinus surgery merits investigation due to the risk of cerebrospinal fluid (CSF) leak as a result of intra-operative damage to the cribriform plate. A sample of rhinorrhoea may be tested for the presence of β2-transferrin, which is almost 100% specific for the presence of CSF. In a child presenting with a history of unilateral purulent nasal discharge there should be a high index of suspicion of foreign body. Allergic rhinitis causes sneezing, rhinorrhoea and nasal blockage, and may be associated with conjunctivitis. It may be seasonal or perennial depending upon the nature of the allergen.

16. Answers: 1C 2F

The American Joint Committee on Cancer/UICC staging system for laryngeal carcinoma is used in the UK. Vocal cord movement should be normal in all T1 cancers. T1a involves one vocal cord, whereas T1b involves both vocal cords. A T2 tumour involves extension to the supraglottis and/or subglottis and/or impaired vocal cord mobility. A T3 tumour is limited to the larynx, but there is a fixed vocal cord. A T4 tumour is associated with invasion of structures outside the larynx.

17. Hoarse voice:

A Chronic laryngitis
B Vocal cord nodules
C Vocal fold polyps
D Carcinoma of the vocal cord
E Vocal cord palsy
F Reinke's oedema
G Vocal cord granuloma
H Oesophageal carcinoma
I Fibrosing alveolitis

For each of the following scenarios, select the most likely pathology:
1 A 35-year-old woman complains of persistent hoarseness. She has a previous history of multiple ITU admissions for brittle asthma.
2 A 45-year-old advertising consultant presents with hoarseness. He is a non-smoker. Nasendoscopy reveals symmetrical ovoid lesions on the anterior third of the vocal folds.

18. Acute stridor:

A Inhaled foreign body
B Respiratory papillomatosis
C Chronic obstructive airways disease
D Tracheo-oesophageal fistula
E Acute laryngotracheobronchitis (croup)
F Anaphylactic reaction
G Pharyngitis
H Acute epiglottitis
I Acute tonsillitis
J Asthma

For each of the following scenarios, select the most likely cause:
1 A 2-year-old child presents with a 24-hour history of cough and stridor following a recent flu-like illness. On examination the child looks comfortable and is mildly pyrexial.
2 A 3-year-old boy presents with rapid onset of noisy breathing and drooling. On examination the child is pyrexial, appears distressed and has marked stridor.

17.   Answers: 1G 2B

Vocal cord granulomas result from chronic irritation or trauma. Prolonged or repeated endotracheal intubation is a risk factor for granuloma formation. Treatment depends upon the cause, but anti-reflux therapy and voice therapy are generally indicated to increase the speed of recovery. Vocal fold nodules are typically located at the junction of the anterior and middle two-thirds of the vocal fold, where contact is most forceful. They most commonly occur in patients with a history of excessive voice use or vocal abuse. Treatment with speech therapy is usually curative, but some patients may require surgical excision.

18.   Answers: 1E 2H

Acute laryngo-tracheobronchitis is a viral inflammation of the upper respiratory tract (most commonly a parainfluenza virus) that can lead to upper airway obstruction. It is associated with the clinical sign of a barking cough. The disease is often mild and self-limiting, and resolves without any active intervention. However, significant progressive inflammation and subglottic swelling, especially around the level of the cricoid cartilage, can lead to life-threatening airway obstruction. Acute epiglottitis is a medical emergency caused by inflammation and severe oedema of the epiglottis. Initial symptoms include rapidly progressive severe sore throat associated with dysphagia and high fever. Swelling of the epiglottis and supraglottic structures causing stridor and breathing difficulty may develop rapidly.

19. Throat pain:

A Pharyngeal candidiasis

B Quinsy

C Chronic tonsillitis

D Infectious mononucleosis

E Tonsillitis

F Squamous-cell carcinoma of the tonsil

G Vestibular schwannoma (acoustic neuroma)

H Vocal cord nodule

I Foreign body

For each of the following clinical scenarios, select the most likely diagnosis:

1 A 16-year-old student presents with a 5-day history of lethargy, malaise and increasing throat pain. She is unable to eat, and can only drink small sips of water. On examination both tonsils are enlarged and inflamed with a white exudate on the surface. There is marked bilateral cervical lymphadenopathy. Full blood count shows a lymphocytosis.

2 A 62-year-old smoker presents with a 3-week history of left-sided throat soreness and pain on swallowing. He has also noticed some pain in the ear.

3 A 40-year-old man presents with a 4-day history of worsening throat pain that is worse on the left side. He is unable to eat or drink, and has noticed a change in his voice. On examination, he has difficulty opening his mouth, tonsil inflammation and soft palate swelling on the right side. The uvula is deviated to the left.

20. Sinus anatomy:

A Supra-orbital cell

B Anterior ethmoidal cell

C Posterior ethmoidal cell

D Maxillary sinus

E Uncinate process

F Frontal sinus

G Concha bullosa

H Infra-orbital cell

I Sphenoid sinus

J Agger nasi

K Suprabullar recess

Select the appropriate anatomical structure for each of the following descriptions:

1 Cells medial to the lamina papyracea that drain into the middle meatus.

2 A pneumatised middle turbinate.

19.   Answers: 1D 2F 3B

Primary Epstein–Barr virus (EBV) infection causes infectious mononucleosis (glandular fever). The patient presents with non-specific symptoms including fever, lethargy, malaise and lymphadenopathy. The tonsillitis may be associated with tonsillar hypertrophy that causes significant oropharyngeal obstruction. The tonsils are characteristically coated with a white exudate, and there may be petechial haemorrhages over the hard palate. Cervical lymphadenopathy is prominent. Full blood count shows a lymphocytosis (neutrophilia is seen in bacterial tonsillitis). The Paul–Bunnell antibody test is used to confirm the diagnosis, but a negative result does not preclude the diagnosis of infectious mononucleosis in the context of a clinical picture of EBV infection. Throat pain with odynophagia in the absence of infection requires urgent investigation. Referred pain to the ear is also suggestive of malignancy. Peritonsillar abscess (quinsy) may complicate a severe tonsillitis, and presents with sore throat, dysphagia and the classic 'hot-potato' voice. Examination reveals a peritonsillar bulge causing deviation of the uvula to one side. Treatment involves aspiration or incision and drainage together with antibiotic therapy.

20.   Answers: 1B 2G

The ethmoidal cells lie medial to the lamina papyracea that forms the medial orbital wall. The anterior ethmoidal cells drain into the middle meatus, whereas the posterior ethmoidal cells (posterior to the ground lamella of the middle turbinate) drain into the superior meatus. A pneumatised turbinate is termed a concha bullosa and occurs in around 10% of people. It almost always involves the middle turbinate.

21. Airway management:

A Guedel airway
B Nasopharyngeal airway
C Endotracheal intubation
D Needle cricothyroidotomy

F Tracheostomy
G Laryngeal mask airway
H Face mask
I Distraction osteogenesis

For each of the following clinical scenarios, select the appropriate airway management technique:

1 A 3-week-old boy is diagnosed with Pierre Robin sequence. He is struggling to breathe despite repeated repositioning.

2 A 53-year-old man is due to undergo a left modified radical neck dissection, jaw-split and hemi-glossectomy for an extensive tongue and oral carcinoma.

22. Rhinitis:

A Seasonal allergic rhinitis
B Perennial allergic rhinitis
C Vasomotor rhinitis

D Hormonal rhinitis

E Atrophic rhinitis
F Occupational rhinitis
G Non-allergic rhinitis and eosinophilia syndrome
H Rhinitis medicamentosa

For each of the following clinical scenarios, select the most likely diagnosis:

1 A 68-year-old woman presents with severe foul-smelling crusting in the nose. She has previously been successfully treated with radiotherapy for sinonasal carcinoma.

2 A 23-year-old woman who is 6 weeks pregnant presents with new symptoms of clear rhinorrhoea and nasal obstruction.

21.   Answers: 1B 2F

A nasopharyngeal airway is the most appropriate initial management for cases of Pierre Robin sequence that fail conservative management. This will overcome the tongue base obstruction to the airway that accompanies the mandibular hypoplasia of Pierre Robin sequence. Tracheostomy is an alternative if nasopharyngeal intubation fails. In the second scenario an elective temporary tracheostomy is the norm. The post-operative swelling of the tongue base needs to be overcome for the first few post-operative days.

22.   Answers: 1E 2D

Atrophic rhinitis is a rare abnormality that occurs when the normal ciliated mucosa of the nasal cavity is replaced with squamous cells. This can occur as a primary disorder or secondary to surgery, radiation, trauma or infection. There is a characteristic overwhelming foul smell due to infected crusts in the nose, although the patient has lost olfactory capacity and so is unaware of this. Rhinitis can occur at any point during pregnancy, but usually occurs in the first trimester. It affects 20% of pregnancies, and the cause is uncertain, but may be related to placental growth hormone.

23. Epistaxis:

A Hereditary haemorrhagic telangiectasia   E Nasal polyps

B Wegener's granulomatosis   F Pyogenic granuloma

C Syphilis   G Inverted papilloma

D Foreign body   H Leukaemia

Select the most likely diagnosis for each of the following scenarios:

1 A 41-year-old woman presents with painful crusting and epistaxis. She suffers from shortness of breath at rest and renal impairment. Chest X-ray shows multiple cavitating lesions. Urinalysis shows haematuria.

2 A 35-year-old man presents with mild recurrent epistaxis. Anterior rhinoscopy shows a smooth red swelling of the nasal septum.

23. Answers: 1B 2F

ENT involvement in Wegener's granulomatosis is a common early manifestation of the disease. Nasal symptoms include nasal obstruction, facial pain and epistaxis. Involvement of the nasal septum can result in septal perforation and external deformities such as saddle-nose. Wegener's granulomatosis is associated with a glomerulonephritis that may lead to renal failure. Urinalysis may show proteinuria and haematuria. Biopsy of affected lesions is the gold standard for diagnosis. There is an association of Wegener's granulomatosis with a positive cANCA result (95% specific, but much less sensitive). Pyogenic granuloma is a misonomer for a capillary haemangioma that typically arises at sites of trauma or chronic irritation; the lesion is not pyogenic and is not a granuloma. Typically early lesions are vascular and appear as smooth pink or red swellings.

Head and neck

24. Neck dissection:

A Radical neck dissection
B Modified radical neck dissection
C Supraomohyoid neck dissection

D Lateral neck dissection
E Posterolateral neck dissection
F Anterior neck dissection

Match each of the following descriptions to the correct type of neck dissection:

1 Removal of lymph nodes in levels I–V, the spinal accessory nerve, the sternomastoid muscle and the internal jugular vein.
2 Removal of lymph nodes in groups I–III.

25. Dysphagia:

A Foreign body
B Pharyngeal pouch
C Mallory–Weiss syndrome
D Globus pharyngeus

E Post-cricoid carcinoma
F Oesophageal atresia
G Diffuse oesophageal spasm
H Oesophageal achalasia

For each of the following clinical scenarios, select the most likely cause:

1 A 68-year-old man complains of regurgitation of food and halitosis. He has been treated with courses of antibiotics for recurrent chest infections.
2 A 55-year-old woman complains of a 3-month history of throat pain and progressively worsening difficulty with swallowing. Full blood count reveals iron-deficiency anaemia.
3 A 35-year-old woman describes a long history of dysphagia and cramping pains in the chest. Barium swallow reveals a dilated tapering oesophagus.

24. Answers: 1A 2C

Neck dissection is the removal of lymphatic tissue from the neck. Radical neck dissection includes removal of the spinal accessory nerve, the sterno-mastoid muscle and the internal jugular vein; all other neck dissections are a modified radical neck dissection. Selective neck dissections remove only certain lymphatic groups (levels I–III in a supraomohyoid dissection, levels II–IV in a lateral neck dissection, levels II–V in a posterolateral dissection, and level VI in an anterior dissection).

25. Answers: 1B 2E 3H

Regurgitation of food, a reducible lump in the neck, recurrent chest infections and halitosis are all features of a pharyngeal pouch. The combination of odynophagia (pain on swallowing) and dysphagia are red flags for malignancy that merit urgent investigation. Oesophageal achalasia is associated with a failure of relaxation of the lower oesophageal sphincter, and may present with symptoms of dysphagia, regurgitation and chest pain. Barium swallow shows the typical finding of a dilated tapering oesophagus. Oesophageal manometry may also be useful in establishing the diagnosis.

26. Paediatric neck masses:
    A Lymphoma   E Sternomastoid tumour
    B Thyroglossal cyst   F Branchial cyst
    C Cervical rib   G Abscess
    D Lymphatic malformation H Lipoma
       (cystic hygroma)

For each of the following scenarios, select the most likely diagnosis:
1 A 6-year-old child presents with a 1 cm spherical firm midline swelling below the hyoid bone. The child's mother reports that in the past it has been inflamed, but that it has improved with oral antibiotics.
2 A 7-year-old girl presenting with a history of night sweats and weight loss is found to have multiple non-tender smooth masses on both sides of the neck.
3 A 2-year-old child presents with a soft compressible mass in the right posterior triangle which is noted to have brilliant translucency.

27. Management of thyroid masses:
    A Total thyroidectomy   F Hemithyroidectomy and
                                     chemotherapy
    B Hemithyroidectomy and   G Radiotherapy
       radiotherapy
    C Sistrunk's procedure   H No further treatment
    D Excision biopsy and   I Hemithyroidectomy
       radiotherapy
    E Radio-iodine ablation   J Chemotherapy

For each of the following scenarios, select the appropriate treatment strategy:
1 A 42-year-old woman presents with a left-sided thyroid lump. Fine-needle aspiration shows a Thy3 follicular lesion.
2 A 9-year-old boy complains of a midline cystic neck swelling which moves upward on tongue protrusion.
3 A 32-year-old patient presents with a 3 cm left-sided thyroid lump. A left thyroid lobectomy is performed, and the histology report describes a follicular adenoma.

26.   Answers: 1B 2A 3D

A thyroglossal cyst is classically situated at or just alongside the midline, and moves with protrusion of the tongue. Infection should be treated with antibiotics, and incision and drainage should be avoided as there is a risk of sinus formation. Once the infection has completely resolved, excision via Sistrunk's procedure is the treatment of choice. This involves an en bloc resection including the cyst and body of hyoid, and following any tract to the tongue base and thyroid isthmus. Fever, night sweats and weight loss are known as B symptoms, and are associated with non-Hodgkin's lymphoma. Although non-specific, the presence of B symptoms with lymphadenopathy should arouse suspicion of lymphoma. A soft compressible mass in the posterior triangle may be a lipoma but, particularly in view of the presence of brilliant translucency, a lymphatic malformation should be considered as more likely.

27.   Answers: 1I 2C 3H

A Thy 3 result suggests a follicular lesion/follicular neoplasm. As a distinction cannot be made between follicular adenoma and carcinoma with fine-needle aspiration cytology alone, hemithyroidectomy is required for diagnosis. Sistrunk's procedure is the surgery of choice for excision of a thyroglossal cyst, and has a much lower rate of recurrence compared with excision of the cyst alone. Follicular adenoma is a benign lesion, and therefore excision of the lesion by lobectomy is sufficient treatment.

28. Adult neck masses:

A Thyroid nodule
B Cervical rib
C Lipoma
D Lymphoma
E Pharyngeal pouch

F Branchial cyst
G Plunging ranula
H Pleomorphic adenoma
I Chemodectoma
J Submandibular lymph node

For each of the following scenarios, select the most likely diagnosis:

1 A 34-year-old woman complains of a firm swelling at the base of the right posterior triangle associated with some weakness of the muscles of the right hand.

2 A 30-year-old man presents with a smooth, non-tender, fluctuant mass along the upper one-third of the anteromedial border of the sternocleidomastoid muscle between the muscle and the overlying skin. He reports that it became inflamed a few years ago but responded to a short course of oral antibiotics.

3 A 52-year-old man presents with a smooth pulsatile mass below the angle of the jaw.

29. Nerves of the head and neck:

A Glossopharyngeal nerve
B Accessory nerve
C Brachial plexus
D Inferior alveolar nerve
E Facial nerve
F Lingual nerve

G Chorda tympani
H Lesser auricular nerve
I Superior laryngeal nerve
J Hypoglossal nerve
K Abducent nerve

For each of the following functions, choose the appropriate nerve:

1 Supplies motor innervation to the posterior belly of the digastric muscle.

2 Supplies taste and general sensation to the posterior third of the tongue.

3 Supplies motor innervation to the sternocleidomastoid muscle.

28. Answers: 1B 2F 3I

A cervical rib may present as a bony mass in the root of the neck. It may cause a form of thoracic outlet syndrome by compression of branches of the brachial plexus or subclavian artery. The typical position for a branchial cyst is at the junction of the lower two-thirds and upper one-third of the sternocleidomastoid muscle. If there is a history of cigarette smoking or if the lesion presents after the age of 40 years, the possibility that this is actually a cystic neck metastasis should be considered. A pulsatile mass should raise suspicion of an aneurysm (if it is expansile) or a carotid body tumour (chemodectoma). Classically a chemodectoma is not mobile vertically but is mobile laterally due to its adventitial attachments. Investigation for any excessive catecholamine production is important, particularly if surgical excision is planned. As a rule of thumb, 10% of tumours are malignant, 10% are familial and 10% secrete catecholamines.

29. Answers: 1E 2A 3B

The facial nerve exits the stylomastoid foramen and gives off several branches before it enters the parotid gland. These branches include the posterior auricular nerve and a muscular branch supplying the occipital belly of the occipitofrontalis, the stylohyoid and the posterior belly of the digastric muscle. The posterior third of the tongue receives sensory and taste fibres from the glossopharyngeal nerve. The anterior two-thirds receive sensory fibres from the lingual nerve (mandibular branch of V) and taste fibres from the chorda tympani (VII). The accessory nerve supplies the sternomastoid and trapezius muscles.

30. Nerve injuries in head and neck surgery:

A Lingual nerve   F Vagus nerve
B Accessory nerve   G Recurrent laryngeal nerve
C Brachial plexus   H Phrenic nerve
D Glossopharyngeal nerve   I Superior laryngeal nerve
E Marginal mandibular   J Great auricular nerve
   nerve

For each of the following scenarios, select the nerve that is most likely to have been injured:

1 A 44-year-old patient is found to have drooping of the lower lip following parotidectomy.
2 A 33-year-old patient complains of numbness of the anterior part of the tongue following submandibular gland excision.
3 A 44-year-old patient has some difficulty in shrugging his right shoulder following a modified radical neck dissection.

31. Complications of head and neck surgery:

A Glossopharyngeal nerve   G Recurrent laryngeal nerve
   injury   injury
B Accessory nerve injury   H Lingual nerve injury
C Brachial plexus injury   I Superior laryngeal nerve
                                      injury
D Frey syndrome   J Great auricular nerve injury
E Reflex sympathetic   K Hypoglossal nerve injury
   dystrophy
F Marginal mandibular   L External laryngeal nerve
   nerve injury   injury

For each of the following scenarios, select the most likely complication:

1 A 34-year-old patient reports sweating over the cheek during mealtimes following a superficial parotidectomy.
2 A 26-year-old patient reports some hoarseness of the voice following right hemi-thyroidectomy. Nasendoscopy reveals a right-sided vocal cord palsy.
3 A 44-year-old patient is found to have fasciculation over the right side of the tongue several months after removal of the right submandibular gland.

30.   Answers: 1E 2A 3B

All branches of the facial nerve within the parotid gland are at risk during parotidectomy. Injury to the marginal mandibular nerve may result in disfiguring drooping of the lower lip. There is potential for injury to the lingual, hypoglossal and marginal mandibular nerves during submandibular gland surgery. Difficulty in shrugging the shoulder post neck dissection implies injury/intentional sacrifice of the accessory nerve.

31.   Answers: 1D 2G 3K

Gustatory sweating (sweating during eating) is the classic feature of Frey syndrome. The auriculotemporal nerve carries sympathetic fibres to the sweat glands and parasympathetic fibres to the parotid gland. It is hypothesised that following surgery, section of these nerves and abnormal re-innervation results in the phenomenon of gustatory sweating. Injury to the recurrent laryngeal nerve is a risk associated with thyroidectomy, and may result in vocal cord palsy. Hypoglossal nerve injury may result in fasciculation and weakness of the affected side of the tongue.

32. Vessels of the head and neck:

A Superior thyroid vein

B Anterior jugular vein

C Lingual artery

D Internal jugular vein

E Occipital artery

F Facial vein

G Maxillary artery

H External jugular vein

I Superior thyroid artery

J Innominate artery

K Internal carotid artery

L Ascending pharyngeal artery

Select the appropriate vessel from each of the following anatomical descriptions:

1 Formed by the union of the posterior auricular vein and the retromandibular vein.

2 First branch of the external carotid artery.

33. Salivary gland tumours:

A Oncocytoma

B Adenolymphoma (Warthin's tumour)

C Acinic-cell carcinoma

D Adenoid cystic carcinoma

E Ductal papilloma

F Pleomorphic adenoma

G Mucoepidermoid carcinoma

H Malignant melanoma

Match the correct diagnosis to each of the following descriptions:

1 A benign mixed tumour composed of epithelial and myoepithelial cells in a stroma.

2 A slow-growing malignancy that typically grows along nerve sheaths.

32.   Answers: 1H 2L

The external jugular vein is formed by the union of the posterior division of the facial vein with the posterior auricular vein. It therefore receives the majority of blood from the exterior of the cranium and deep parts of the face. The external carotid artery extends from the bifurcation of the common carotid artery to the midpoint of the mastoid process and angle of mandible. It initially lies antero-medial to the internal carotid artery, and has several branches (unlike the latter). These branches include the superior thyroid, lingual, facial, occipital, posterior auricular and ascending pharyngeal branches. The external carotid artery finally bifurcates to give rise to the maxillary and superficial temporal arteries.

33.   Answers: 1F 2D

Pleomorphic adenoma is the most common tumour of the salivary gland, and is so called because it is composed of epithelial and connective tissue components. It typically occurs in the tail of the parotid gland. Adenoid cystic carcinoma is the most common malignancy of minor salivary glands, but also occurs in the major salivary glands. Impalpable lesions in the parotid may present with progressive facial palsy due to the capacity of the tumour to invade nerve sheaths.

34. Skull foramina:
    A Foramen magnum
    B Jugular foramen
    C Foramen lacerum
    D Foramen ovale
    E Foramen rotundum
    F Stylomastoid foramen
    G Foramen spinosum
    H Condylar canal

    Select the foramen through which each of the following structures exits the cranium:
    1 Vagus nerve.
    2 Maxillary (V2) nerve.

35. Staging of head and neck cancer:
    A T2 N2 M0
    B T4 N3 Mx
    C T3 N2b Mx
    D T1 N2a Mx
    E T3 N3 Mx
    F T2 N1 Mx
    G T1 N1 Mx
    H T2 N3 Mx

    For each of the following tumours, select the appropriate TNM stage:
    1 A 45-year-old woman presents with a right-sided hard irregular parotid lump. MRI shows a 3 cm tumour with a 2 cm right level I lymph node.
    2 Panendoscopy of a 65-year-old man with odynophagia reveals a 2 cm exophytic lesion of the left piriform fossa with a fixed left vocal fold. MRI scan identifies two 2.5 cm lymph nodes in the right level II area of the neck.

34. Answers: 1B 2E

The jugular foramen provides passage to the sigmoid sinus (becoming the internal jugular vein upon exiting the skull) and the glossopharyngeal, vagus and accessory nerves. The foramen rotundum is the exit point for the maxillary nerve.

35. Answers: 1F 2C

Parotid tumour staging follows the AJCC/UICC TNM classification system (T1, tumour < 2 cm; T2, tumour 2–4 cm without extraparenchymal extension; T3, extraparenchymal extension and/or tumour 4–6 cm; T4, invasion of facial nerve and/or tumour > 6 cm). The left piriform fossa tumour is invading the hemilarynx, causing a fixed vocal fold, and so is classified as T3. The presence of multiple ipsilateral lymph nodes < 6 cm classifies the nodal stage as N2b (N0, no lymph nodes; N1, single node < 3 cm; N2a, a single ipsilateral node 3–6 cm; N2b, multiple ipsilateral nodes < 6 cm; N2c, bilateral or contralateral nodes < 6 cm; N3, node > 6 cm).

Miscellaneous

36. Surgical complications:
    A 100%   D < 50%
    B 10%   E < 0.1%
    C 1%

    Select the most appropriate surgical complication rate for each of
    the following procedures:
    1 Return to theatre for haemorrhage following tonsillectomy.
    2 Optic nerve injury following antrostomy and anterior ethmoid-
      ectomy.
    3 Dead ear following stapedotomy.
    4 Vocal cord palsy following a level I neck dissection.

37. Paediatric airway:
    A Laryngomalacia   E Acquired subglottic stenosis
    B Tracheo-oesophageal fistula F Vocal cord palsy
    C Asthma   G Laryngeal web
    D Bilateral choanal atresia

    For each of the following clinical scenarios, select the probable
    cause of paediatric breathing difficulties:
    1 Inspiratory stridor developing in a 6-week-old child.
    2 A 3-month-old child has a history of gradual onset of stridor.
      The child was born prematurely at 22 weeks' gestation and was
      ventilated for 6 weeks.
    3 A 9-month-old child has a history of repeated episodes of
      pneumonia.
    4 An 11-month-old child has undergone cardiac surgery and has
      now developed hoarseness.

36. Answers: 1C 2E 3C 4E

At least 3% of patients will bleed following tonsillectomy, and 1% will need to return to theatre for bleeding to be stopped. Injury to the optic nerve is rare during sinus surgery, and this nerve is anatomically only at risk during surgery to the posterior sinuses, not the anterior ones. Dead ear may occur following routine stapedotomy in around 1% of cases, and is thought to be due to perilymph leak. The recurrent laryngeal nerve is not anatomically at risk during a level I neck dissection.

37. Answers: 1A 2E 3B 4F

Laryngomalacia typically develops at 6 weeks of age. Inspiratory stridor occurs due to lack of rigidity of supraglottic structures, and it can be treated expectantly in almost all cases. Endotracheal intubation is associated with a risk of development of subglottic stenosis, and is therefore especially common in ex-premature children who require prolonged ventilation due to respiratory immaturity. Tracheo-oesophageal fistula may present with recurrent pneumonia or choking episodes during feeding. The thoracic portion of the left recurrent laryngeal nerve is at risk during cardiothoracic surgery, and may present with stridor and hoarseness.

38. Cranial nerve function:

A Abducent nerve (VI)

B Facial (VII) nerve

C Glossopharyngeal (IX) nerve

D Vagus (X) nerve

E Vagus (X) recurrent laryngeal branch

F Accessory (XI) nerve

G Hypoglossal (XII) nerve

H C1 nerve fibres

Select the appropriate cranial nerve for each of the following functions:

1 Secretomotor fibres to the parotid gland.

2 Taste to the anterior two-thirds of the tongue.

3 Sensation to the middle ear.

39. Classes of immunoglobulin:

A IgA

B IgD

C IgE

D IgG

E IgM

Match the correct immunoglobulin class to each of the following inflammatory processes:

1 Seasonal allergic rhinitis.

2 Autoimmune Graves disease.

38. Answers: 1C 2B 3C

The glossopharyngeal nerve exits the skull through the jugular foramen, and shortly gives off a branch that enters back up into the middle ear. This branch supplies sensory fibres to the middle ear and some fibres that re-enter the cranium as the lesser petrosal nerve. The lesser petrosal nerve exits the cranium again to synapse in the otic ganglion and supply secretomotor fibres to the parotid gland. Taste fibres to the anterior two-thirds of the tongue are carried on the facial nerve, which gives off the chorda tympani in the middle ear to traverse the tympanic cavity and join the lingual nerve to the tongue.

39. Answers: 1C 2D

Seasonal allergic rhinitis is a type 1 hypersensitivity reaction to pollen that is mediated through IgE release from, for example, mast cells. Graves disease of the thyroid is caused by an IgG auto-antibody that stimulates the TSH receptor.

40. Thyroid cytology:

A Thy 0   E Thy 4
B Thy 1   F Thy 5
C Thy 2   G Thy 6
D Thy 3

For each of the following results on fine-needle aspiration, select the appropriate cytological classification:

1 A 42-year-old woman presents with a well-circumscribed right-sided thyroid lump. The fine-needle aspiration sample is bloodstained and inadequate for interpretation.
2 A 26-year-old patient presents with a 2 cm right-sided thyroid cystic lesion. Fine-needle aspiration shows features suggestive of a colloid nodule with the presence of benign epithelial cells.
3 A 45-year-old man presents with a 3 cm right thyroid nodule. Fine-needle aspiration shows unequivocal features of papillary carcinoma.

41. Pharyngeal (branchial) arches:

A First pharyngeal arch   G First pharyngeal pouch
B Second pharyngeal arch   H Second pharyngeal pouch
C Third pharyngeal arch   I Third pharyngeal pouch
D Fourth pharyngeal arch   J Fourth pharyngeal pouch
E Fifth pharyngeal arch   K Fifth pharyngeal pouch
F Sixth pharyngeal arch

For each of the following structures, select the correct embryological origin:

1 The stapes.
2 The superior parathyroid glands.
3 The palatine tonsil.
4 The glossopharyngeal nerve.
5 The tensor tympani muscle.

40. Answers: 1B 2C 3F

The Thy classification obtained by analysis of FNAC samples along with a detailed text report may be useful in the planning of surgery. The diagnosis of malignancy cannot always be made by FNAC alone. The broad interpretation of the Thy classification is as follows: Thy 1, inadequate; Thy 2, non-neoplastic; Thy 3, follicular lesion/suspected follicular neoplasm; Thy 4, suspicious of malignancy; Thy 5, diagnostic of malignancy.

41. Answers: 1B 2J 3I 4C 5A

Each pharyngeal arch contains a cartilage, muscle, artery and nerve component. The first pharyngeal arch includes the malleus, incus zygoma, mandible (cartilage), mylohyoid, tensor tympani and palati and the muscles of mastication (muscle), maxillary artery and mandibular branch V nerve (artery and nerve). The second arch includes the stapes, styloid, upper half and lesser cornu hyoid bone (cartilage), stapedius, stylohyoid, posterior belly of digastric (muscle), facial nerve and stapedial artery (nerve and artery). The third arch gives rise to the greater cornu hyoid, stylopharyngeus, common carotid artery and glossopharyngeal nerve. Remember that the inferior parathyroids develop from the third pouch and the superior parathyroids develop from the fourth pouch (the third pouch develops faster and becomes shifted caudally during development).

42. Management of foreign bodies:
    A Heimlich manoeuvre
    B EUA of the nose and removal
    C Oesophagoscopy and removal
    D Removal with parental restraint
    E Regular backslaps
    F Alternating chest/abdominal thrusts
    G Rigid bronchoscopy and removal
    H IV fluids, buscopan and observe
    I No treatment required

    For each of the following scenarios, select the most appropriate management strategy:
    1 A 5-year-old child with learning difficulties presents with an offensive unilateral purulent discharge from the right nostril.
    2 A 25-year-old woman is referred to the ENT team after complaining of suspected food bolus obstruction. She was eating some steak 2 hours ago and swallowed a bolus without chewing it properly. She is swallowing her own saliva but regurgitates large sips of water. She is uncomfortable but not in distress.
    3 A 4-year-old girl is brought to the emergency department after her parent suspected that her daughter had inhaled a peanut. Chest X-ray shows a collapsed right lung.

43. Radiological imaging:
    A Ultrasound scan
    B CT scan
    C MRI scan
    D PET scan
    E Radio-nuclide scanning
    F Angiography
    G Plain X-ray

    Select the most appropriate imaging technique for each of the following investigations:
    1 Assessment of the extent of middle-ear cholesteatoma.
    2 Preliminary imaging of an asymptomatic thyroid nodule.

42. Answers: 1B 2H 3G

A foreign body should always be considered when there is presentation of unilateral foul-smelling discharge in a child. Some foreign bodies may be removed with a compliant patient and parent, but often an examination under anaesthesia is required to minimise the risk of causing nasal trauma. A boneless meat bolus obstruction may be managed conservatively with intravenous fluids and buscopan in the first instance if the patient is not distressed. Inhaled foreign bodies that have caused lung collapse in a child require bronchoscopic removal under a general anaesthetic, preferably with the presence of a paediatric anaesthetist.

43. Answers: 1B 2A

CT is the best modality for pre-operative imaging of the extent of chole-steatoma, as it will demonstrate bony erosion into structures such as the semicircular canals, cochlea or middle cranial fossa. Thyroid nodules are best assessed by ultrasound, which will show their consistency, homo-geneity, margin and blood flow. Some authors question the value of any imaging of thyroid nodules, but ultrasonographic demonstration of doppler blood flow is showing promise as a predictive tool for malignancy, and ultrasound-guided fine-needle aspiration cytology is more accurate than that without radiological guidance.

44. Microbial pathogens:

A Herpes simplex virus
B Epstein–Barr virus
C Human papilloma virus
D Rhinovirus
E Respiratory syncytial virus

F *Staphylococcus aureus*
G *Streptococcus pneumoniae*
H *Haemophilus influenzae*
I *Corynebacterium diphtheriae*
J *Candida albicans*

For each of the following disorders, identify the most commonly associated microbial pathogen:

1 Epiglottitis.
2 Nasopharyngeal carcinoma.

45. Complications of infection:

A Bezold's abscess
B Ramsay Hunt syndrome
C Meningo-encephalitis
D Retropharyngeal abscess

E Lateral sinus thrombosis
F Citelli's abscess
G Subdural abscess
H Gradenigo syndrome

For each of the following clinical scenarios, select the appropriate complication of infection:

1 A 6-year-old child presents with severe otalgia and a discharging left ear. On examination he is distressed with a pyrexia and tenderness over the mastoid. CT shows a subperiosteal collection spreading through the medial aspect of the mastoid into the digastric fossa.

2 A 5-year-old child has been treated with oral antibiotics for acute tonsillitis. He is brought to the emergency department acutely distressed with fever, drooling, mild stridor and significant bilateral cervical lymphadenopathy. There is severe trismus and the child is reluctant to move his head from side to side.

44.   Answers: 1H 2B

Epiglottitis is typically caused by *Haemophilus influenzae* type B, and its incidence has rapidly declined due to vaccination against this bacterial serotype. Streptococcus, varicella or candida can also cause this disease, albeit less frequently. Epstein–Barr virus, and antibodies to it, are consistently found in the majority of patients with nasopharyngeal carcinoma, and the virus is listed as a recognised carcinogen.

45.   Answers: 1F 2D

Following severe acute otitis media, pus in the middle ear and mastoid cells may erode through the bone overlying the mastoid to form a collection in the subcutaneous tissues. Occasionally the infection may track along subcutaneous tissues into the neck. If the infection tracks down the digastric groove and along the fascial plane of the sternomastoid sheath, it can form an abscess within the substance of the muscle (Bezold's abscess). Citelli's abscess refers to infection that has spread through the medial aspect of the mastoid into the digastric fossa. This may result in osteomyelitis of the occipital bone. Retropharyngeal abscess may be a complication of a severe tonsillitis with accompanying suppuration of retropharyngeal nodes. The child may present in a similar fashion to an acute epiglottitis, with drooling and the neck held rigidly or hyperextended. There may be signs of acute airway obstruction with stertor and stridor. An inspiratory lateral soft tissue radiograph will show widening of the retropharyngeal space. Treatment involves close airway observation, administration of intravenous antibiotics, and incision and drainage via an external approach under general anaesthetic.

46. ENT manifestations of systemic disorders:

A Systemic lupus erythematosus	F Relapsing polychondritis
B Wegener's granulomatosis	G Ehlers–Danlos syndrome
C Syphilis	H Churg–Strauss syndrome
D Rheumatoid arthritis	I Reiter syndrome
E Ankylosing spondylitis	J Sarcoidosis

For each of the following scenarios, select the most likely diagnosis:
1 A 55-year-old African man complains of a purplish raised lesion over the right alar rim. On examination, bilateral cervical lymphadenopathy is found. Blood tests show hypercalcaemia.
2 A 60-year-old woman is found to have significant collapse of the bony nasal septum. There is no history of previous trauma or surgery.

47. Surgical incisions:

A Modified Blair incision	E Caldwell–Luc incision
B MacFee incision	F Lynch–Howarth incision
C Post-auricular incision	G Bi-coronal flap
D McBurney incision	H Lateral canthotomy

For each of the following procedures, select the most appropriate incision:
1 External ethmoidectomy.
2 Superficial parotidectomy.

46. Answers: 1J 2C

Lupus pernio is a characteristic cutaneous lesion of sarcoidosis. It has a high predictive value for involvement of the lungs and sites in the ear, nose and throat. The lesion is typically red or purple, and may be associated with shiny skin changes. It is sarcoid specific, and is more common in individuals of African origin and in women. Tertiary syphilis occurs several years after the initial infection, and is characterised by the deposition of granulomata (known as gummas) at any site in the body. Gumma deposition in the bony nasal septum may cause depression and collapse of the nasal bridge to leave a saddle-nose deformity. Although rare, syphilis should always be considered in the context of bony septal erosion in the absence of trauma or previous surgery.

47. Answers: 1F 2A

The Lynch–Howarth incision is an incision vertically along the lateral nasal bones and curving around along the inferior border of the supra-orbital ridge. It is used in external ethmoidectomy, and also to gain access to the frontal sinus. A modified Blair incision begins in front of and just above the tragus, curves down behind the lobule and then follows along the anterior border of the sternomastoid muscle. It affords a broad base for exposure of the parotid gland.

48. Statistical terms:

A *P*-value   F Mode

B Standard deviation   G Mean

C Inter-quartile range   H Range

D Median   I Incidence

E Prevalence   J Power

For each of the following descriptions, select the appropriate statistical term:

1 The most frequent observation in a data set.

2 The difference between the smallest and largest values in a data set.

49. Endocrine function:

A Thyroid epithelial (follicular) cells   E Oxyphil cells of the parathyroid gland

B Parafollicular (C) cells of the thyroid   F Carotid body glomus cells

C Chief cells of the parathyroid gland   G Chromaffin cells of the adrenal medulla

D Renal cells   H Neurosecretory cells of the anterior pituitary

For each of the following functions, select the appropriate cell type:

1 Secretion of thyroid hormone.

2 Secretion of calcitonin.

48. Answers: 1F 2H

There are several tests of the average value in a data set. The mean is the sum of all values divided by the number of values. The median is the middle of all values when they are listed in size order. The mode is the most frequent value. The range describes the difference between the largest and smallest value.

49. Answers: 1A 2B

Thyroid hormone (T3 and T4) is excreted by the follicular epithelial cells of the thyroid gland. Calcitonin reduces serum calcium levels and is also released from the thyroid gland (the parafollicular cells). Its effect is countered by parathyroid hormone released from the chief cells of the parathyroid gland, which raises serum calcium levels.

50. Post-operative investigations:

A Echocardiography

B Chest X-ray

C ECG

D MRI

E PET

F Ventilation-perfusion scan

G Twenty-four-hour blood pressure monitor

H Serum calcium

For each of the following scenarios, select the most useful investigation:

1 A 45-year-old man complains of the sudden onset of right-sided pleuritic chest pain 4 days post-laryngectomy.

2 A 34-year-old woman complains of tingling in the fingers on the first post-operative day following total thyroidectomy.

50. Answers: 1F 2H

There is significant risk of deep vein thrombosis and pulmonary embolus following surgery, due to factors relating to dehydration and immobility. Ventilation–perfusion scan or CT pulmonary angiogram are the investigations of choice. Efforts are made to preserve the parathyroid glands during total thyroidectomy. However, there is still a risk of hypocalcaemia post-operatively. Mild hypocalcaemia may be treated with oral supplementation, but severe hypocalcaemia should be treated with intravenous calcium gluconate to minimise the risk of life-threatening cardiac arrhythmia.

Index

accessory nerve 153/154; 155/156
acoustic neuroma 11/12
acute mastoiditis 131/132
acute suppurative otitis media 5/6; 7/8; 17/18; 21/22
adenocarcinoma
    follicular 75/76
    papillary 75/76
    pleomorphic 77/78
adenoid cystic carcinoma 157/158
adenoidectomy 35/36
adenolymphoma 71/72
airway management
    adult 143/144
    paediatric 163/164
allergic rhinitis 35/36; 45/46
    investigations 47/48
    seasonal 109/110; 137/138; 165/166
    severe 113/114
Alport syndrome 125/126
anaesthetics, local 103/104
anaplastic carcinoma, thyroid 77/78
angiofibroma 37/38; 85/86
anosmia 55/56
    causes 41/42; 47/48
antibiotics, ototoxic 13/14
antrochoanal polyp 135/136
argon laser 55/56
Arnold–Chiari malformation 47/48
Arnold's nerve 25/26
atrophic rhinitis 143/144
audiometry 123/124
    objective vs. subjective tests 31/32
    see also individual tests
auditory brainstem implants 125/126

aural atresia, congenital 19/20
autoimmune diseases 109/110

bacterial pathogens 171/172
BAHAs *see* bone-anchored hearing aids (BAHAs) 29/30
balance tests 27/28
Barrett's oesophagus 91/92
basal-cell carcinoma 101/102
bat ear deformity 101/102
Bell's palsy 71/72
benign paroxysmal positional vertigo (BPPV) 9/10; 19/20; 123/124
Bezold's abscess 171/172
Blair incisions 173/174
blood volume, infants 111/112
bone-anchored hearing aids (BAHAs) 29/30; 129/130
brainstem electrical response audiometry 31/32
branchial arches 167/168
branchial (pharyngeal) cysts 93/94
Brown–Sequard syndrome 89/90
Budd–Chiari syndrome 47/48

calcitonin 93/94; 175/176
caloric testing 27/28
carotid artery rupture 83/84
cauliflower ear deformity 101/102
cerebrospinal fluid rhinorrhoea 43/44; 137/138
cetuximab 111/112
Charcot–Marie–Tooth disease 61/62
CHARGE syndrome 35/36

chemotherapeutic drugs 13/14; 111/112
Chi-squared test 105/106
choanal atresia 35/36
cholesteatoma 9/10
    surgery 27/28
chylous fistula 79/80
cigarette smoking 99/100
cilia 49/50
cisplatin 111/112
Citelli's abscess 171/172
cleft palate 19/20; 63/64
clinical trials 115/116
cochlea
    anatomical features 17/18
    measurement of function 23/24
Cogan syndrome 61/62
concha bullosa 141/142
conductive hearing loss, causes 7/8; 17/18; 29/30; 31/32; 121/122
congenital aural atresia 19/20
congenital stridor 39/40
consent issues 105/108
Cotton grading system 37/38; 83/84
cranial nerve function 165/166
croup 139/140
Crouzon syndrome 51/53; 61/62
CT scans 115/116; 169/170
cystic hygroma 151/152
cytomegalovirus 17/18

dizziness investigations 123/124
Down syndrome 115/116
drug toxicity 13/14
dysphagia 149/150

Eagle syndrome 109/110

ear discharge, treatments 131/132
ear wax 29/30
electronystagmography 27/28
endocrine function 175/176
endotracheal intubation 81/82; 163/164
epiglottitis 171/172
epistaxis 57/58
  causes and risk factors 37/38; 45/46; 51/54; 145/146
  control measures 135/136
Epworth Sleepiness Scale 99/100
ethmoidal cells 141/142
ethmoidectomy 173/174
eustachian tube, anatomical features 27/28
evidence-based medicine (EBM) 103/104
exostoses 29/30
external carotid artery 67/68
external jugular vein 157/158

facial haemangiomas 81/82
facial nerve 153/154; 165/166
  branches 65/66
  malformations 19/20
facial nerve palsy 21/22
  causes 61/62
  complications 71/72
facial plastics 113/114
Factor V Leiden 45/46
fine-needle aspiration cytology (FNAC) 99/100
fistula
  chylous 79/80
  perilymph 25/26
  tracheo-oesophageal 163/164
follicular adenocarcinoma 75/76
foramen rotundum 159/160
foreign bodies
  ear 29/30
  management 169/170
  nose 137/138
fragile X syndrome 61/62
Frey syndrome 47/48; 71/72; 155/156
frontal sinus 51/53

Gaussian (normal) distribution 105/106
glandular fever 109/110

glomus tumour 131/132
glossopharyngeal nerve 89/90; 153/154; 165/166
Graves disease 87/88
great auricular nerve 25/26
grommets, complications 15/16
Guillain–Barré syndrome 77/78

haemangiomas, facial 81/82
haematoma, complications 101/102
head and neck cancers
  see laryngopharyngeal carcinomas
head and neck nerves 153/154; 165/166
  post-surgery complications 155/156
head and neck vessels 157/158
hearing aids 129/130
  bone-anchored (BAHAs) 29/30; 129/130
hearing loss
  causes 7/8; 17/18; 11/12; 29/30; 121/122; 125/126
  conductive 7/8; 17/18; 29/30; 31/32; 121/122
  congenital 129/130
  noise-induced 11/12
  sensorineural 31/32; 121/122
  syndromic 125/126; 129/130
  treatments 125/126
hearing measurement
  general considerations 7/8; 15/16; 31/32
  objective vs. subjective tests 31/32
  see also individual tests
hereditary haemorrhagic telangiectasia 51/54
hoarse voice 139/140
holoprosencephaly 41/42
human papilloma virus (HPV) 41/42
hypoglossal nerve 75/76; 87/88
  injury 155/156
hypopharyngeal carcinoma 73/74
hypovolaemic shock 111/112

imaging 115/116; 169/170; 177/178

immunoglobulins 165/166
in-the-canal hearing aid 129/130
infants 111/112; 151/152
infectious mononucleosis 141/142
infratemporal fossa 89/90
Isshiki thyroplasty 37/38; 47/48

Jerger tympanogram classifications 23/24
Jervell and Lange–Nielsen syndrome 125/126
jugular foramen 159/160
juvenile angiofibroma 37/38; 85/86

Kallmann syndrome 41/42
Kartagener syndrome 49/50
keratosis obturans 28/29
Keros classification system 43/44
Kiesselbach's plexus 57/58; 135/136

laryngeal carcinoma 41/42; 51/52; 137/138
laryngeal cartilages 43/44
laryngeal nerve injury 155/156
laryngeal surgery 55/56; 177/178
laryngo-tracheobronchitis 139/140
laryngocoele 51/52
laryngomalacia 39/40; 163/164
laryngopharyngeal carcinomas 109/110
  staging 159/160
laser surgery 97/98
lignocaine 103/104
lingual nerve 73/74; 155/156
Little's area 57/58; 135/136
local anaesthetics 103/104
Ludwig's angina 91/92
lupus pernio 173/174
Lyme disease 61/62
lymphatic malformations 65/66
lymphoma 151/152
Lynch–Howarth incision 173/174

malignant melanoma 97/98
malignant otitis externa 21/22

Mann–Whitney test 105/106
marginal mandibular nerve 155/156
mastoid process 23/24
  surgery 21/22; 27/28
mastoidectomy 21/22
maxillary hyperostosis 61/62
melanoma 97/98
melphalan 111/112
Ménière disease 7/8; 31/32; 123/124
middle ear, tympanometry 23/24
Moebius syndrome 19/20
Mondini dysplasia 17/18; 25/26
motile cilia 49/50
MRI scans 115/116
multiple endocrine neoplasia (MEN) 101/102
myoclonus, palatal 19/20
myringoplasty 21/22
myringosclerosis 17/18

nasal obstruction 135/136
nasal polyps 43/44; 135/136
nasal sprays, overuse 135/136
nasal tamponade 57/58
nasal trauma, septal perforation 39/40
nasolacrimal duct 49/50
nasopharyngeal angiofibroma 37/38; 85/86
nasopharyngeal carcinoma 17/18; 171/172
neck
  anatomical features 69/70; 71/72
  injuries 89/90
  masses 75/76; 77/78; 93/94; 151/152; 153/154
  surgery 83/84; 149/150
neonatal hearing investigations 23/24
nerve injuries, post-surgery 155/156
noise-induced hearing loss 11/12
nose bleeds see epistaxis
nystagmus 15/16

obstructive sleep apnoea 99/100
oesophageal achalasia 149/150
oesophageal carcinoma, squamous cell 101/102

oesophageal perforation 69/70
oesophagoscopy, complications 69/70
olfactory nerve, damage 41/42; 55/56
optic nerve 37/38
oral cavity carcinoma 73/74
oral leucoplakia 87/88
orbital blow-out fractures 109/110
orbital cellulitis 63/64
Osler–Weber–Rendu syndrome 45/46
osteogenesis imperfecta 17/18
osteomas 29/30
osteosclerosis 5/6; 31/32; 121/122
otalgia 13/14; 127/128
  causes 29/30
  complications 171/172
  treatments 131/132
otitis externa
  causes 11/12
  malignant 21/22
otitis media
  acute suppurative 5/6; 7/8; 17/18; 21/22
  treatments 35/36
otoacoustic emissions (OAEs) 23/24; 31/32; 123/124
ototoxic drugs 13/14

paediatrics 111/112; 151/152
papillary adenocarcinoma, of thyroid 75/76
parathyroid glands 93/94
parotid pleomorphic adenoma 67/68
parotid surgery 77/78; 173/174
Paterson–Brown-Kelly syndrome 73/74; 101/102
pathogens 171/172
patient consent 105/108
Pendred syndrome 125/126
perforated tympanic membrane 21/22; 25/26
perilymph fistula 25/26
peritonsillar abscess 141/142
Pfeiffer syndrome 61/62
pharyngeal arches 167/168
pharyngeal pouch 85/86; 149/150
Pierre Robin sequence 61/62; 129/130; 143/144

pinna
  functions 9/10
  sensory supply 25/26
play audiograms 123/124
pleomorphic adenomas 77/78; 157/158
Plummer–Vinson syndrome 73/74; 101/102
Polly beak deformity 47/48
polychondritis, relapsing 37/38
polycythaemia vera 45/46
post-cricoid carcinoma 149/150
Pott disease 51/53
presbycusis 31/32; 121/122; 131/132
pterygoid plate 65/66
pterygopalatine fossa 85/86
pure-tone audiograms (PTA) 15/16; 31/32; 123/124
pyogenic granuloma 145/146

quinsy 141/142

radio-allergosorbent test (RAST) 47/48
radiological imaging, see also imaging
radiotherapy, complications 81/82
Ramsay Hunt syndrome 71/72; 127/128
recurrent laryngeal nerve 57/58
Reinke's oedema 49/50; 55/56
relapsing polychondritis 101/102; 109/110
respiratory papillomatosis 41/42
retropharyngeal abscess 171/172
Reye syndrome 111/112
rhinitis 35/36; 45/46; 109/110; 143/144
  investigations 47/48
  medicamentosa 135/136
rhinorrhoea 137/138
  cerebrospinal fluid (CSF) 43/44
Rinne test 31/32; 127/128

saccharin test 49/50
saddle-nose deformity 101/102
salivary calculi 91/92

Samter's triad 43/44
sarcoidosis 173/174
Schirmer test 85/86
sensorineural hearing loss, causes 31/32; 121/122
septal haematoma 55/56
septal perforation 39/40
septoplasty, complications 47/48
sinonasal tumours 39/40
sinus, anatomical features 141/142
Sistrunk's procedure 63/64; 151/152
Sjögren syndrome 85–6
skull foramina 159/160
sleep apnoea
    childhood 35/36
    obstructive 99/100
smell disorders 41/42; 47/48; 55/56
smoking 99/100
speech audiometry 31/32
sphenoid sinus, anatomical features 37/8
statistical tests, Gaussian (normal) distribution 105/106
Stenger test 7/8
steroid treatments 113/114
Stickler syndrome 63/64
stridor, acute 139/140
styloid process 23/24; 109/110
subglottic stenosis 37/38
submandibular gland 73/74
surgical complications (general) 163/164
surgical incisions 173/174
surgical sutures 105/107
sutures 105/107
syphilis 173/174

tears 49/50
temporal bone
    anatomical structures 23/24
    fractures 19/20
    infection 21/22
temporal lobe epilepsy 55/56

temporo-mandibular joint (TMJ) 67/68
throat pain investigations 141/142
Thy classification system 167/168
thyroglossal cyst 63/64; 151/152
thyroid
    anatomical features 91/92
    investigations 167/168
thyroid cancer
    adenocarcinoma 75/76
    anaplastic carcinoma 77/78
    management 151/152
    risk factors 77/78
thyroid eye disease 87/88; 109/110
thyroid hormone 175/176
thyroid storm 81/82
thyroidectomy 177/178
tinnitus 19/20; 131/132
tongue, anatomical features 75/76
tonsillectomy 61/62
tonsillitis, severe 141/142; 171/172
tonsils, squamous cell carcinoma 141/142
tracheo-oesophageal fistula 163/164
tracheomalacia 83/84
tracheostomy 143/144
    complications 77/78
    indications 77/78; 143/144
Treacher–Collins syndrome 19/20; 99/100
trigeminal nerve 69/70
    branches 83/84
tuning fork tests 31/32; 127/128
tympanic membrane
    anatomical features 13/14
    calcium deposition (myringosclerosis) 17/18

perforation 21/22; 25/26
    repair 21/22
    retraction of pars tensa 5/6
tympanometry 23/24; 31/32
tympanosclerosis 17/18

ultrasound 115/116; 169/170
Unterberger test 27/28
UPSIT scores 55/56
Usher syndrome 129/130

ventilation tubes, installation complications 15/16
vertigo
    benign paroxysmal positional (BPPV) 9/10
    Ménière disease 7/8; 31/32; 123/124
vestibular function 27/28
vestibular schwannoma 11/12; 31/32; 123/124
video-fluoroscopy 115/116
Vidian nerve 37/38
vincristine 111/112
vocal cord granuloma 139/140
vocal cord nodules 45/46; 139/140
vocal cord palsy 47/48; 163/164

Waardenburg syndrome 125/126
Warthin's tumour 71/72
wax impaction 29/30
Weber test 127/128
Wegener's granulomatosis 113/114; 145/146
Wilcoxon test 105/106
wound healing 103/104

Young's procedure 51/54

Z-plasty 113/114
Zenker's diverticulum 85/86
zygomatic process 23/24

Lightning Source UK Ltd.
Milton Keynes UK
UKHW040135100119
335307UK00008BA/272/P

9 781846 193347